Natural Remedies
from the
Chinese Cupboard

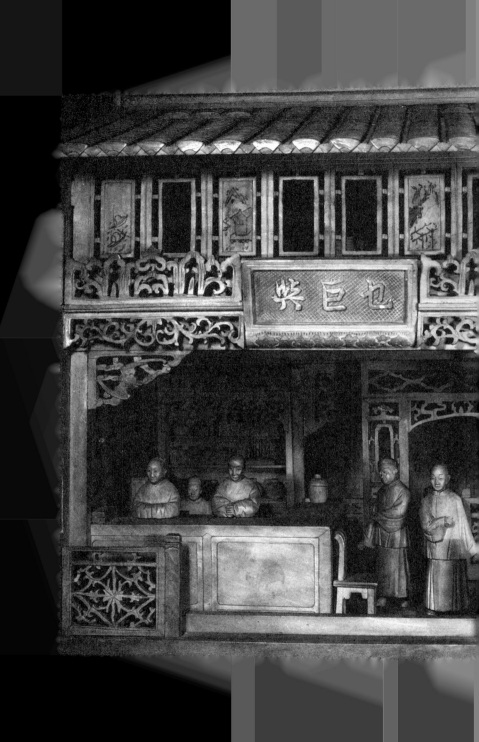

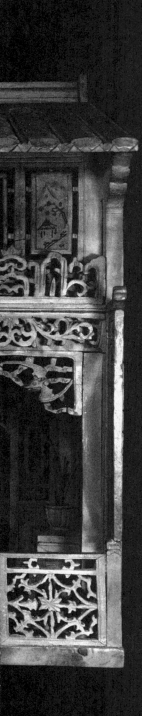

Natural Remedies
from the
Chinese Cupboard

Healing Foods and Herbs

by Dr. Fang Jing Pei

Weatherhill
New York & Tokyo

Cover photo by the author shows a nineteenth-century boxwood model of a traditional Chinese apothecary, from the Ji Zhen Zhai collection.

First edition, 1998

Published by Weatherhill, Inc., of New York and Tokyo. Protected by copyright under the terms of the International Copyright Union; all rights reserved. Except for fair use in book reviews, no part of this book may be reproduced for any reason by any means, including any method of photographic reproduction, without the written permission of Weatherhill, Inc.

Library of Congress Cataloging-in-Publication Data

Fang, Jing Pei
    Natural remedies from the Chinese cupboard: healing foods and herbs / by Fang Jing Pei.—1st ed.
        p. cm.
    ISBN 0-8348-0459-x
    1. Herbs—Therapeutic use. 2. Food, Natural—Therapeutic use. 3. Medicine, Chinese. I. Title.
RM666.H33F365 1998
615'.321'0951–dc21   98-34671
                                                                     CIP

Contents

INDEX OF HERBS

Preface

In this age of rapid and continuing breakthroughs in medical science, including new pharmaceuticals, surgical procedures, medical appliances, and genetic discoveries, it seems remarkable that the interest in alternative medicine, particularly natural food remedies and Chinese herbal medicine, is unusually strong. Those interested include not only people who suffer from chronic ailments or diseases that have no known cure in Western medicine, but also patients who are tired of taking medications with dangerous and debilitating side effects, known and unknown. Physicians as well are looking for answers to intractable medical questions that may lead them into areas in which which they have not been trained. Acupuncture, for example, long recognized in Asia as beneficial for numerous maladies, was unknown in the West until the latter part of this century; now many Western physicians are seeking specialized training in order to to be able to give treatments. The search for alternative treatment methods has produced the realization that therapies suitable for a whole host of human ailments, some of which have been known for thousands of years, are in fact available outside of mainstream Western medical pratice.

My general medical training and specialized training in psychiatry was followed by practice for over twenty-five years. Over the years, I was also exposed to the use of natural food remedies and Chinese herbal medicines by practitioners, colleagues, family members, and friends, both in this country and in China, who have used both therapies throughout their lives and professional practices. Their reasons for doing so were varied. In most instances, those who were exposed at an early age to alternative medical treatments such as natural food cures, accepted them unquestioningly as efficacious treatments passed down from generation to generation, a kind of folk wisdom. Natural food remedies in many cases were like old family friend, commonly known and used without really understanding the mechanisms of their effectiveness. Ginkgo, for instance, has been used for hundreds of years in China for circulatory disturbances. Only recently has the West discovered that the chemical substance in ginkgo indeed has beneficial effects on the circulatory system and may stem the progression of Alzheimer's. The same is true of the ordinary herbs ginger and garlic. However, it isn't necessary to know this to appreciate the usefulness of a traditional remedy and apply it. Most practitioners have been guided by the simple logic of "if it works why not?" while others believe that herbal remedies are more "natural" and so using them is better than introducing synthetic chemical medicines into the body.

Although the philosophical foundations of Chinese medicine and herbal treatments are, as would be expected, markedly different from those of Western medicine, and the terminology daunting (although certainly no more than Western medical jargon!), the basic concepts and relationships are compellingly sensible. In this book, I have attempted to present the basic philosophy behind Chinese herbal medicine in order to provide some understanding of the principles behind the recommended treatments. However, I do not believe it is absolutely necessary that one study or understand these principles. I have also tried to present a "bridge" between Western and Eastern thought in the treatment presentations. These are not meant to replace the proper physical examinations and subsequent treatment recommendations of physicians. Whether readers choose to visit physicians trained in traditional Western or traditional Chinese medicine, a medical consultation is mandatory before embarking on any course of treatment.

This book is not, and was never intended to be, a comprehensive sourcebook of Chinese traditional medical treatments; rather, it has been designed to present only the most common ailments and selected remedies. The clinical picture of each ailment is first presented and the most common symptoms for each described. Natural food remedies are then given; these should be of interest to those who prefer to try first the most "natural" treatment or to those who prefer not to use stronger medications or herbal concoctions. The simplest recipes for preparing the natural food remedies are given, restricted where possible to items readily available in the West.

Next, under Chinese herbal remedies, the "King" herb(s) that would be prescribed for the ailment by practitioners of Chinese herbal medicine are identified, with brief notes on the rationale for their selection. These are followed by brief descriptions of the pharmacological actions of the herbs according to Western medical studies; it is interesting to note the many similarities between the two explanations. Introduction of the King herbs is followed, in most cases, by herbal formulas that would typically be prescribed for the ailment. And since Chinese herbalists might not recognize these herbs from their Western *pinyin* spellings, the Chinese characters have been listed in an index.

If nothing else, my own studies of both traditional Western medicine and Chinese herbal medicine have proved to me that there are often multiple solutions to medical problems, including some outside of those offered by Western medicine. Moreover, sometimes where one normally efficacious treatment fails, another works. Both patients and medical professionals with open minds should realize that the best solutions to medical problems may thus include a combination of traditional and alternative therapies.

This publication is not intended to encourage self-treatment. It is rather a reference work based upon the observations of the author, a medical professional, and discussions with physicians in China who practice Chinese herbal medicine; it was designed to show differences in the practice of traditional Chinese medicine and Western medicine and, in some instances, underlying similarities. It was further intended to introduce to the reader natural food remedies, so called "household treatments" that have proved beneficial for many generations. If you feel that a treatment identified herein might be appropriate for you, it should only be instituted under the guidance of your physician. Self-diagnosis and treatment is dangerous and not recommended under any circumstances.

Traditional Chinese Medicine

Traditional Chinese Medicine

Medicine is the art and science of healing disease. Yet, the practice of medicine in China and the West take very different approaches to their common goal. Although appreciated for its descriptive detail and philosophical syncretism, Chinese traditional medicine has not been, until recently, respected for its treatment methods. Indeed, in the not too distant past any positive effects of traditional Chinese medicine were viewed as the result simply of a placebo effect; the patient thought he was getting better and therefore felt better. Acupuncture, herbal medicine, and *qi gong* (activities design to cultivate and project *qi*, often translated "intrinsic energy") were all viewed as having little relevance to scientific treatment. Acupuncture and *qi gong*, in particular, were looked upon as something just short of witchcraft.

Yet during the past decade, there has been immense reawakening of interest in these traditional Chinese therapies. Although *qi gong*, a healing practice said to utilize the healing qi energy of the therapist directed through the main acupuncture points of his body, and thereby effecting the qi flow of the patient, remains mysterious with respect to its mechanisms, we currently find many Western practitioners trained in the principles of acupuncture, which is now utilized by many respected practitioners as an accepted therapeutic technique. Likewise, many herbs utilized in traditional herbal medicine have since been studied and found to have positive effects for specific disorders. In ailments where there have been no specific remedies, in a search to find a cure or treatment, many have turned to Chinese herbal medicine to learn how a particular disorder would be treated in China.

CHINESE MEDICAL THEORY

Chinese medicine is based on the theory that disease and illness have their origins in the disturbed emotions of the individual. To the Western physician, emotional disturbances are seen as a discreet type of disorder which may or may not have an effect on the body, but all illnesses are not seen as having origins in emotional illness. Related to this interconnectedness of the physical and the emotional, Chinese medicine approaches illness and its treatment from a holistic perspective. When a malady is present, the total body is seen as being disturbed and warranting treatment; to the Western physician, one speaks of diseased organs rather than the diseased body. Thus the Chinese physician prescribes treatment according to a complex of symptoms that presents itself, while the Western physician prescribes on the basis of the specific organ found to be diseased. These differences may not seem so great; however, the principles and resulting treatments that derive from them have indeed created two very different medical traditions.

Let us first explore some basic terms and concepts to gain an understanding of the way that the Chinese physician views illness and the medical treatment of it, keeping in mind that while these terms and concepts may sound odd or unscientific, they have been used for thousands of years and millions of people have responded to treatments based on them. In any case, we should dismiss the idea that we must choose between Western and Chinese systems, or seek to state equivocally that one method is right and one method is wrong. Indeed, in modern China today, Western and Chinese traditional medicine are both practiced, in some cases side by side and enhancing each other; Western medicine would be best served by exhibiting the same open-mindedness.

YIN AND YANG

The most basic concept of Chinese medicine is that of yin and yang, which in turn exemplify the principle of mutually dependent opposites. In the Chinese world view, yang is associated with heaven, the male sex, brightness, lightness, dryness, the sun, and odd numbers, etc., while yin is associated with the earth, the female sex, darkness, heaviness, dampness, the moon, and even numbers. All things, objective and subjective, are believed have complementary opposites and, therefore all things contain yin and yang aspects. Moreover, these things, whether actual or conceptual, are mutually dependent: "up" has no meaning without the understanding of "down;" "hot" becomes meaningful only when one understands "cold", etc. One can not exist without the other.

Moreover, the relationship is a dynamic interaction; the sun rises to its apogee and then sets; the moon appears when the sun disappears; when the yin of winter ebbs to its greatest degree, the world begins warming to reach the yang of high summer. This concept is seen to pervade all of nature and all phenonmenon and objects in the universe, including man and the structure and workings of the human body. While the total body is seen as a whole structure, the body is divided into yin and yang aspects in the following way:

YIN	YANG
Below the waist	Above the waist
Interior of body	Exterior of body
Front of the body	Back of the body
Middle of the body	Sides of the body
Organs	Organs
Spleen	Small intestine
Heart	Large intestine
Liver	Gallbladder
Lungs	Bladder
Kidneys	Stomach
	San jiao ("triple warmer")

YIN AND YANG BALANCE

The body attempts to maintain a natural balance between yin and yang. Eating, necessary for subsistence, is considered yin while the actions of the body itself, movement which expends energy, is considered yang. Under normal conditions, when one is without illness, the body is said to be in yin and yang balance. Under circumstances that are abnormal, i.e., when the balance is disrupted, there is an excess or lacking of either yin or yang, and a disease process is in evidence. Even the disrupted balance is dynamic and subject to changes. For example, if you have a virus and develop a high fever, the Chinese therapist would say that you have a yang syndrome. But if that fever is suddenly lowered rapidly (for instance, by placing the body in cold water or drinking cool liquids) and the temperature falls below normal so you feel chilled, the disease complex has now changed. The Chinese physician would say that the yang syndrome has changed to a yin syndrome. It is the disruption between the relative balance between yin and yang that results in a pathologic change. The complex interrelationship and interdependence can be summarized as follows:

1. If a disease is caused by yin pathogenesis, yin functioning is disrupted and is hypoactive, which causes injury to yang. This results in a so-called cold syndrome.

2. If a disease is caused by yang pathogenesis, yang functioning is disrupted and is hypoactive, which causes injury to yin. This results in a so-called heat syndrome.

3. However, when yang is deficient it can fail to restrict yin, causing a deficiency *xu*, which results in a cold syndrome.

4. Similarly, a yin deficiency leading to a yang excess can result in a *xu* heat syndrome. Thus,

Yin excess ⟶ cold syndrome
Yang excess ⟶ heat syndrome
Yin deficiency ⟶ heat syndrome
Yang deficiency ⟶ cold syndrome

FUNDAMENTAL TREATMENT CONCEPT

With the basic understanding of the goal of yin and yang balance, treatments are devised to restore balance where imbalance, equivalent to disease, is manifested. The following simplified example illustrates the basic concept of treatment:

A person with pneumonia runs a high fever and has pathogenic heat, a yang disease agent. In this instance, yin becomes deficient to the high degree of present yang. This heat syndrome's treatment will be treated with cold-natured herbs to overcome the heat generated. The cardinal rule is that **yang diseases require yin treatment and yin diseases require yang treatment.**

THE FIVE ELEMENTS

The theory of "five elements" is a Taoist philosophical construct designed to describe and explain nature and its phenomenon. Each of the five elements—wood, fire, earth, metal, and water—have characteristics which correspond to the natural world, including the human body, as well as fixed modes of interrelating with each other. These observed correspondences and known patterns of interrelationship are important in making diagnoses and prescribing treatments.

The table on the following page identifies the organs and qualities corresponding to the five elements. Examining the table, we see that all of the elements have specific characteristics and correspond to specific body parts, organs, tissues, senses, and even directions, colors, seasons, and so on. For example, wood is related to spring, the color blue-green, and, in terms of the human body, the liver and the emotion anger. Water is related to winter, the kidney and the ear, and has the quality of being salty.

Besides illustrating the interrelationships between the five elements and other specific items and attributes, the table also shows us, through its horizontal flow, correspondences between those items and attributes, specifically between body parts and organs. For instance, among the yin organs, the liver supports the heart, the heart supports the spleen, the spleen supports the lungs, the lungs support the kidneys. The kidneys, in turn, support the liver.

In the well person, that is to say the person whose body is in yin-yang balance, the support chain described above would be operative. However, if that person had a diseased spleen, the balanced interrelationship would be disrupted, although it could perhaps be restored if the heart energy was enhanced. When an organ is dis-

7

Five Elements Table

Element	Wood	Fire	Earth	Metal	Water
Season	Spring	Summer	Late Summer	Autumn	Winter
Direction	East	South	Center	West	North
Color	Blue-green	Red	Yellow-orange	White	Black
Climate	Wind	Heat	Damp	Dry	Cold
Taste	Sour	Bitter	Sweet	Pungent	Salty
Smell	Rancid	Burnt	Fragrant	Rotting	Putrid
Yin Organ	Liver	Heart	Spleen	Lungs	Kidney
Yang Organ	Gallbladder	Small intestine	Stomach	Large intestine	Bladder
Orifice	Eyes	Tongue	Mouth	Nose	Ears
Tissue	Tendons	Blood vessels	Muscles	Skin	Bones
Emotion	Anger	Joy	Pensiveness	Grief	Fear
Voice	Shout	Laugh	Sing	Weep	Groan

eased, the equilibrium between all of the elements is disrupted to some degree. Thus, to the practitioner of Chinese traditional medicine, the resultant imbalance can be seen in symptoms exhibited elsewhere than the element initiating the imbalance.

QI AND ITS DISORDERS

Like yin and yang, qi is a concept fundamental to Chinese traditional medicine and has no counterpart in Western medicine. Sometimes translated "intrinsic energy," it is the essential motive energy of all life and activity. It it the "life force," circulating through the body and animating it, actuating its motions and functions. Qi is involved in all movements of the body, in energy entering and leaving the body, and is dynamic. It is also involved in normalizing the body temperature, and as such protects the body from the external influences that may affect body temperature, such as heat, cold, dampness, dryness, etc. Qi, so to speak, is both the programmer of the functioning of the other organs of the body and is involved in the transmission of food and air into substances that nurture the body; it is an agent as well as an actuator. Its chief disorders are described as follows:

1. *Stagnant qi* is blocked or does not flow normally. Swelling in an organ can be an example of stagnant qi.

2. *Deficient qi* is not available or unable to carry out qi functions. An example of qi deficiency is the body's inability to maintain normal temperature, a function of qi.

3. *Sinking qi* is not able to perform its function of holding or supporting the organs; uterine prolapse is an example of sinking qi.

4. *Rebellious qi* flows in the wrong direction. A manifestation of this condition would be vomiting.

Blood in Chinese medicine is, not surprisingly, viewed differently than in the West. It is closely associated with qi and, in fact, is a product of qi. By the action of qi moving the blood, blood provides nourishment, the nutritive mechanism of qi. As well, it provides moisture and lubrication to the body and the nutriments required for clear thinking. There are three chief disorders of the blood: stagnant blood, deficient blood, and heat in the blood. Stagnant blood is seen as not moving in sufficient quantity or strength. Associated with this disorder are cancerous growths, pain, and swelling. Deficient blood is caused by a lack of production of blood, leading to related disorders as well as dryness. Lastly, heat in the blood leads to emotional problems and disorders related to the liver.

BODY FLUIDS

In addition to blood, body fluids provide the moisture, lubrication, and nourishment to all areas of the body. There are two types of body fluids, clear and dense. The clear fluids are controlled by the lungs and moisten external components of the body—muscles, skin, hair, eyes, ears, mouth, nose, etc. Dense fluids are controlled by the spleen and kidneys and circulate through the interior of the body, providing nourishment to the joints and brain. Disorders of body fluids are of two types: deficient body fluids or accumulation of body fluids. Deficient body fluids can result in dry skin disorders, constipation, etc., while accumulations of body fluids can result in swelling, pneumonia, and similar problems.

CAUSES OF ILLNESS

We have noted the importance that Chinese traditional medicine places on balance and harmony, and its corollary view of illness as a disruption of harmony, a disruption of equilibrium, a disruption of balance. Disharmony is seen to arise in three areas:

Internal
External
Food, Sex, Energy, and Heredity

Internal The internal causes of illness rest with the disruption of the seven emotions: anger, joy, sadness, grief, pensiveness, fear, and fright. The following table illustrates the relationship between these emotions, the *zang* organs (those associated with yin), and the *fu* organs (associated with yang).

Emotions	Zang Organ	Fu Organ
Anger	Liver	Gallbladder
Joy	Heart	Small Intestine
Sadness, grief	Lungs	Large Intestine
Pensiveness	Spleen	Stomach
Fear, fright	Kidney	Bladder

It should be noted that inherent in the concept of the seven emotions is that all of these emotions are felt by and affect each and every person. However, balance is key to one's emotional, and consequently, physical, health; an excess of any of these is not good. When there is emotional imbalance, disharmony results that may show its symptoms in the zang or fu organs. Looking at the above table, the emotions listed on the left relate to harmony in the corresponding zang and fu organs. However, if there is a disturbance in the emotions resluting in, for example, an overabundance of anger in a person, the liver or the gallbladder might be disturbed, and thus disturbing harmony among the other zang and fu organs. Not only will there be evidence of an overabundance of anger, there will be a corresponding disturbance in the other emotions and organs, as they cannot be in balance. Thus, although the symptoms of this overabundance of anger will likely appear in the liver and gallbladder, they might appear elsewhere as well.

External Wind, cold, dampness, dryness, summer heat, and fire are known as the six external pathogens. Each of these are capable of invading the body through the mouth, nose, or skin causing superficial disease.

Wind is considered a yang pathogen and can act alone or in tandem with another external pathogen. Wind-cold penetration is most common, as in the common cold. Initially, a cold is considered a yin syndrome; however, when fever develops, the symptoms change and it becomes a yang syndrome. Wind can be related to internal disharmony, most often with the liver.

Cold is considered a yin pathogen. Its invasion of the body is rapid, causing the patient to feel cold and experience chills and headache without evidence of sweating or fever. Cold invasion frequently can extend to the lungs, stomach, and spleen as well as the liver.

Dampness, a yin pathogen, and internal dampness is caused by the spleen's inability to function properly, thereby removing dampness as spleen yang is deficient. The most common symptoms are moist appearance, a light pulse, edema, sallow complexion, scant urine, and poor appetite. There may be some swelling of the abdomen.

Fire is a yang pathogen. Fire causes a disturbance in heat, leading to drying and reduced movement. Fever, inflammation, erythema, skin eruptions, dried body fluids, constipation, and scant urine are all in evidence. Fire conditions are usually liver, stomach, lung, and head disturbances.

Summer heat is a yang pathogen causing fever, depression, perspiration, rapid pulse, and headaches. With the reduction in fluids there is fatigue and dryness.

Dryness, a yang pathogen, causes a reduction in yin fluids and can be either internal or external. External dryness causes dry lips dry cough, constipation and pain in the ribs.

Food, Sex, Energy, and Heredity Each of these items plays an important part in the yin-yang balance of the individual, with any imbalance causing a disruption of harmony and affecting related organs. To cite a few examples: Food-related imbalances are most commonly caused by overeating, eating excess foods with cold energy, toxic foods, or and intoxication through drinking. Energy or fatigue is related to working excessively, resulting in a qi deficiency that caused the lungs to function imporperly. Mental fatigue can damage the spleen and cause yin deficiency, while internal fatigue can be caused by overindulgence in sex, causing harm to the kidneys.

In traditional Chinese medical practice, diseases that have been defined according to the above philosophic principles are most often treated with herbs. Herbs have been utilized for treatment dating back to the era of the Three Emperors (2852-2597 B.C.) and there has been considerable documentation of specific herbs throughout China's history. In the Ming Dynasty (1368-1644), the *Compendium of Chinese Medicinal Herbs (Pen tsao kang mu)* noted some 1898 herbs, while the modern *Dictionary of Chinese Herbal Drugs (Chung yao ta tsu tien)* lists some 5,767 drugs, although fewer than 600 are in common use.

Considerable research has been conducted in an effort to identify both the pharmacological effects and the chemical constituents of these drugs. However, despite the vast corpus of information now available on the effects of these compounds, they are still prescribed on the basis of medical theories foreign to the Western physician, namely herbal energies, flavor, movement, and meridian routes. These are briefly introduced below.

The Four Energies Herbs are classified as having four energies: hot, cold, warm, and cool. Based on clinical observation, herbs are divided into those herbs having yin cold and yin cool energy and yang warm and yang hot energy. For example, an herb effective in treating a hot syndrome is considered to have cold energy.

Meridian Routes A meridian route is the path through which an herb enters and travels through the body while exerting its influence. These are important in that although many herbs may be considered to possess the same energy, they make take different paths through the body. Obviously, one would want the herb to travel to the diseased organ to impart its effectiveness.

Five Flavors Herbs are further distinguished by their classification into five flavors: sweet, sour, pungent, bitter, and salty. Each flavor is believed related to specific qualities and felt to impart particular effects. For example, salty herbs promote a downward movement, sour herbs constrict, sweet herbs create harmony, bitter herbs dry, and pungent herbs promote a flow of energy.

Movements As indicated by the example of salty herbs above, herbs are felt to impart movements: upwards, downwards, floating, or sinking. Again, this is particularly important in the choosing of an herb; an herb that pushes downward, for example, could be utilized effectively in the treatment of a cough whose symptom is an upsurging of wind and phlegm.

Action All herbs have specific actions on the body. This concept is readily understood, as Western pharmaceuticals also have specific actions. However, as would be expected, the Chinese terminology for describing these actions is often quite different. Some terms are obvious or self-explanatory, such as counteracting toxic effects, but others are directly related to the basic Chinese traditional medical principles, such as cooling blood, clearing heat, and stopping wind.

PRESCRIBING HERBAL PREPARATIONS

Given the interrealtionships between the organs and parts of the body, and the myriad possible combinations of qualities and effects of the herbs, prescribing herbs or herbal formulas becomes a complex undertaking. The prescribing is based on a thorough clinical evaluation of the patient, taking into account each of the disturbed areas (i.e., the symptoms), which leads to a specific diagnosis. This process is not unlike the Western concept of examining the patient and making a diagnosis. If a patient comes to the Chinese doctor with a nosebleed, the prescribing is done upon determining the cause of the nosebleed, i.e., excessive heat or excessive cold. This information would determine which herb should be prescribed, taking into consideration the meridian utilized by the herb as well as its movement. In the same manner, the Western physician would evaluate the patient and prescribe medication or treatment based on the condition causing the nosebleed.

The prescribing of herbs once a diagnosis has been made is a clinical decision. There are thousands of standard Chinese herbal formulas in addition to special herbal formulas that might be concocted by individual physicians. In most cases, single herbs are not prescribed but rather several herbs are utilized. Most formulas consist of a "king herb," the primary herb responsible for treating the condition, a "subject herb," which assists the king herb by enhancing its effect, an "assistant herb," which treats a minor accompanying symptom, and a "servant herb," which directs the formula to the affected area.

EXPLANATION OF TREATMENT FORMATS

I hope that this brief overview has imparted a sense at least of the complexity and sophisication of China's system of traditional medicine. Obviously, given the myriad realtionships involved in each malady, not to mention the myriad potential combinations of appropriate herbs, the practitioner of this art must undergo decades of study and practice before he or she can be accounted as even moderately skilled. Does that mean that because you have not reached that level of understanding you can not utilize Chinese herbal medicine or natural food remedies? The answer to this question, obviously, is no. You simply need to know that such potentially efficacious remedies exist, then seek out professional opinion as to whether one or more of them might be appropriate for you. The purpose of this book is provide the basic information you will need to discuss these avenues of treatment with a professional.

The text is organized by the most common name of the condition or malady, in alphabetical order. As some of even the most common names of maladies may be unfamiliar, you may need to read further, through the extended definitions and descriptions of symptoms, which are followed by the simplest and most readily available, to my knowledge, natural food remedies. These in turn are followed by a list of the most efficacious Chinese herbs, with a brief description of their actions, and a commonly prescribed herbal preparation. In a few cases, what would be the Chinese herbal remedy may be identical to the natural food remedy; in such cases no separate entry is given for the Chinese herbal remedy. In brief, each entry contains the following:

Title Identifies the ailment by its Western name.

DEFINITION Defines the ailment according to Western terms.

SYMPTOMS The predominant symptoms of the ailment are listed.

NATURAL FOOD REMEDIES

Each natural food remedy mentioned includes a recipe that takes into account availability of required foods in the West and the difficulty of concocting them.

CHINESE HERBAL REMEDIES

Latin names, common names (if available), and Chinese names are given for each key herb used for treating the specified ailment. Chinese names are given in *pinyin*, a romanization system for transcribing Chinese characters according to sound. Since in some instances Chinese pharmacists will not be able to identify the herb by this spelling, an index of all Chinese characters for the herbs listed is included in the back of the book.

The traditional Chinese medical use of each herb is next given, followed by available information regarding the pharmacological action of the herb. Note that in some instances these actions have been studied only through research conducted with animals.

TYPICAL HERBAL FORMULA

Finally, we have seen that traditional Chinese herbs are most often prescribed in formulas containing many herbs. For most maladies listed, a common herbal preparation, with typical quantities and dosages, is given.

Ailments
and Treatments

Alcohol Abuse

DEFINITION An addictive disorder in which there is uncontrolled, excessive alcohol intake. While there are conflicting views as to whether this disorder has psychological origins or biochemical origins, the sufferer drinks in excess, which effects his or her work, emotions, and ability to perform. Left untreated and with continued excessive intake, there are deteriorating effects on the internal organs, which may lead to death.

SYMPTOMS Alcohol intake which results in a desire for increased alcohol intake and dependence both physically and emotionally upon consumption. Common symptoms include early daily drinking, a continued pattern of excessive drinking with dependence on alcohol to control one's nerves, use of alcohol as a tranquilizer, and inability to function without some degree of alcohol intake.

NATURAL FOOD REMEDIES

Kudzu, a plant introduced from Japan to stop soil erosion, has now become a plant of uncontrolled growth in the southern U.S., and is said to grow as much as several inches per hour in prime conditions. Although in the past the plant has had little known herbal use in this country, it has recently been found to have benficial effects on persons who abuse alcohol, acting as an antabuse (a medication which does not allow patients to indulge in substance abuse without experiencing severe nausea and vomiting). When the root extract is infused to make a tea and taken by persons who have problems with alcohol, remarkable effects are observed. Dependence upon alcohol is lessened, the desire to drink is reduced, drinking becomes less uncontrolled, and there is an overall lessening of the severity of depression.

Extract of the root is currently available. Two tablespoons can be infused with four cups of water, with three cups of the liquid taken daily. There have been reports that the dried leaves can also be infused to make a tea which has a similar effect.

Allergies

DEFINITION   An allergic reaction is a hypersensitive state of the body which is acquired by a person upon exposure to a particular allergen(s), such as plants, animal danders, pollution, etc. Upon re-exposure, the body exhibits an altered capacity to react. In simple language, this means that the body is exposed to something to which it is hypersensitive (like breathing in a particular pollen), and when the body is re-exposed to the pollen, its ability to react to this foreign substance is changed. Symptoms can be mild to severe, the severest being an anaphylactic reaction, which is life threatening. Allergies in this section are limited to mild to moderate reactions, e.g., ailments commonly known as hay fever, allergic dermatitis, or rash, allergic sneezing, and the like. In most instances, persons who suffer from allergies (such as hay fever) are aware of the onset of the symptoms, for example, at a particular time of the year, or when they are exposed to a particular animal. Knowing of the allergic material, they are able to act. If you do not know the particular allergen to which you are sensitive, the situation is more problematic. This requires investigation on your part. Think about what new material you have had exposure to. In a process of elimination, you may or may not be able to discover the culprit. You may have to seek medical help. While not being life threatening in most cases, allergies are annoying and disturbing to the point that they may interfere with daily activities and frequently are accompanied by a multitude of mild symptoms. Keep in mind that allergens may not only be animal dander or plant pollen but also can be any foreign items introduced to the body, such as certain foods, food additives, etc.

SYMPTOMS   The most common symptoms are sneezing, headache, coughing, tearing of the eyes, running nose, nosebleeds, itching, rashes, stuffy nose, and reddening of the eyes. Any time you are faced with more severe symptoms such as difficulty in breathing or change in your cardiac status you should seek medical help immediately.

When allergy season is about to arrive, it is important to get a jump on the symptoms which will surely follow. Institute treatment by taking natural food remedies *prior* to the onset of your symptoms. Treatments have found to have greater effectiveness when begun early. While not all remedies are equally effective with all persons, you can probably find a remedy effective for you.

First, try bee pollen. Purchase fresh honey in the comb and cut the honeycomb with its enclosed honey in one inch squares. Chew as you would gum at least three to four times a day.

Plants that provide relief from allergies are members of the allium family, including red onions and scallions, Job's tears, and leafy green vegetables such as spinach, bok choy, Chinese kale, spearmint, basil, and celery. Onions can be processed in a blender with equal amounts of carrots. The juices are then mixed with a small amount of honey to taste. Six ounces should be taken daily.

The seeds of Job's tears can also be made into a natural tea. One teaspoon of seeds are steeped in a cup of hot water for ten minutes and then strained. The very palatable tea can be sweetened with honey or sugar to taste and should be taken at least twice daily. A sprinkling of cinnamon or nutmeg may make this tea more to your liking.

Spinach, spearmint, bok choy, Chinese kale, basil, and celery have all been reported to have positive effects in reducing the symptoms of allergies and should be included in the daily diet. This can be accomplished with salads or as cooked vegetables, although the uncooked vegetables are preferable. In many instances, these vegetables can be combined, blended, and the juices extracted to form a vegetable cocktail. It is advisable to begin by taking 3 ounces a day of the vegetable juices, diluted with another 3 ounces of water, for the first three to four days. Then, at least 6 ounces should be ingested daily.

E<small>FFECTIVE</small> C<small>HINESE</small> H<small>ERBS</small>

Rhei rhizoma • Rhubarb • *Da huang*
Traditionally believed to cool the blood and remove stagnation while dispersing stagnant blood. Pharmacologically, has astringent

and antibacterial effects. In studies with laboratory animals is found to have an anticarcinogenic effect.

Radix ledebouriellae • Siler • *Fang feng*
Traditionally is said to dispel dampness and reduce wind. Pharmacologically, has an antipyretic, antibacterial, and antiviral effect.

TYPICAL HERBAL FORMULA

Rhei rhizoma (Da huang)
Radix ledebouriellae (Fang feng)
Radix angelicae sinesis (Dang gui)
Radix scutellariae (Huang qin)

Alzheimer's Disease

DEFINITION Alzheimer's Disease is a neurologic disorder of the brain whose cause is at present unknown. Once thought of as a rare disease, it is now recognized as one of the common causes of senility. While the condition is not reversible with our current knowledge, it is known that there is marked deterioration of the brain tissue, a reduction in the normal metabolic glucose levels in the brain, and a decrease in the production of brain chemicals. In layman's terms, Alzheimer's Disease is seen as an advanced and rapid case of senility. While sufferers of this disease are not keenly aware of their deterioration, to members of the family or acquaintances, it is emotionally wrenching to watch helplessly the progression of the disease, which can be slow or rapid.

SYMPTOMS The most common symptom of Alzheimer's Disease is memory loss, usually first noticeable in areas with which the sufferer has acute knowledge, such as familiar names, addresses, or the like. With the memory loss there is a delayed response in ordinary situations and at times depression and anxiety. The symptoms rapidly increase and in severe cases there are personality changes and sudden violent episodes. When the illness reaches this degree, the patient may need total care and supervision.

While the disease is considered non-reversible, ginkgo has been shown to delay deterioration and to enable the sufferer to carry on with a normal life for a significantly longer period. The earlier the person is treated with ginkgo the better the response. Ginkgo is available in a variety of forms, including the dry herb as well is in tablet form. In China, a tea or drink is made of the dried leaves, which are simply steeped in boiling water. The dried fruits of the tree are also eaten. However, in both of the previously mentioned forms, it is difficult to regulate the correct daily dosage of 120 milligrams, so the extract form is most conducive to treatment. A response may not be seen for several weeks.

Foods high in B vitamins are felt to have a positive effect as well. These include leafy green vegetables. An effective tonic, 8 ounces of which should be taken daily, are juices extracted equally from Chinese kale, celery, parsley, and bok choy.

EFFECTIVE CHINESE HERBS

Ginkgo semen • Ginkgo • *Yin xing*
Traditionally used to promote qi. Pharmacologically, increases blood flow.

Radix ilicis pubescentis • *Mao dong qing*
Traditionally used to clear heat and resolve toxins. Pharmacologically, improves blood circulation.

Amenorrhea

DEFINITION Amenorrhea is the absence or stoppage of menses, in common terms, an interruption of the female's period. The etiology of this disorder is multifold and can range from disorders of weight (obesity or thinness due to eating disorders), hormonal deficiency, organic disorders, emotional disorders, or any combination of the aforementioned.

SYMPTOMS These may include the complete stoppage of menses or alteration in the flow to below the norm for the individual. The clue to the etiology or cause of this disorder may be found in the secondary symptoms which may accompany the alteration of menses. These could be, among others, change in eating habits, such as undertaking a stringent diet, binge eating, elimination from the diet of greens or meats, emotional turmoil causing depression, anxiety or panic, or other alterations in the body.

NATURAL FOOD REMEDIES

Vitamin intake should be increased by increasing ingestion of fruits and leafy green vegetables. While cooked vegetables are acceptable, the juices and raw vegetables themselves are preferable. Green leafy vegetables such as spinach, Chinese broccoli, Chinese kale, parsley, and coriander can be pulverized with equal amounts of carrots and celery and their juices extracted. Twice daily doses of 8 ounces should be taken.

If there has been alteration in eating patterns, it is imperative for the individual to return to a well-balanced diet that includes the major food groups. Obviously, if the altered dietary habits of the individual have produced symptoms of amenorrhea, the diet is too stringent.

Ginger can be taken either in tablet form or in its natural form. A ginger tea can be prepared by taking two slices of ginger and steeping the slices in two cups of boiling water for five minutes. Strain and sweeten with honey to taste. This ginger tea should be ingested at least twice daily and should replace coffee intake.

Sage is a member of the salvia family that not only has a relaxing effect on the emotions but also relieves spasms of smooth muscle. Sage leaves can be ingested in salads or mixed with other vegetables; however, it is particularly effective as a tea. If fresh sage leaves are utilized, 4 to 5 leaves are steeped in 1 cup of boiling water for 4 to 5 minutes. The leaves will settle to the bottom. Honey can be added to taste and the tea should be ingested at least two to three times daily. If fresh sage leaves are not available, a scant teaspoon of sage can be added to a cup of water and the mixture steeped for five minutes and then filtered.

The herb agnus castus (*Vitex agnus castus*), although not available in fresh form, is available in tablet form and is reported to stimulate the pituitary gland, resulting in a continuation of the natural process of menorrhea. When agnus castus is taken, it is best taken in a pattern similar to the natural menstrual cycle.

The bean of the Ignatia plant, St. Ignatius' bean, is particularly effective for treating uterine spasms as well as amenorrhea. It is available but only in a prepared form and should be taken twice daily, 25 to 35 milliliters in total.

EFFECTIVE CHINESE HERBS

Radix angelicae sinesis • Angelica • *Dang gui*
Traditionally is said to regulate menses while moving blood Pharmacologically, has an effect of increasing metabolism while also causing both stimulating and relaxing of the uterine muscles.

Poria cocos • Hoelen • *Fu ling*
Traditionally is said to remove dampness while promoting diuresis and soothing the inner spirit. Pharmacologically, has a diuretic and tranquilizing effect.

TYPICAL HERBAL FORMULA

Poria cocos (Fu ling) 10 g.
Rhizoma cnidii (Chuan xiong) 6 g.
Radix paeoniae alba (Bai shao) 10 g.
Rhizoma atractylodis (Bai zhu) 10g.
Radix glycyrrhizae (Gan cao) 6 g.
Radix codonopsis (Dang shen) 10 g.
Radix rehmanniae praeparata (Shou di huang) 10 g.
Radix astragali (Huang qi) 10 g.

Anemia

DEFINITION   Anemia is a condition characterized by a deficiency in blood, either quantity or quality. A deficiency in quality could be the amount of hemoglobin or the number of red blood corpuscles or both. In layman's terms, the hemoglobin is the substance within the red corpuscles that carry oxygen in the blood to the organs of the body. If there is a deficiency in either of these substances, the organs of the body suffer from a lack of oxygen.

Causative factors for anemia are numerous. Among them are loss of blood by hemorrhage, spasm of the blood vessels, abnormalities of the red corpuscles, exposure to toxic substances, and dietary deficiencies. The following herbal treatments are directed toward dietary deficiency.

SYMPTOMS   The most common symptom of anemia due to dietary deficiency is fatigue and listlessness. The person generally just feels run down and is usually pale, especially in the gums and exposed membranes of the eyes. Accompanying symptoms are poor appetite, general weakness, shortness of breath, forgetfulness, and anxiety, usually accompanied by depression.

NATURAL FOOD REMEDIES

The remarkable shiitake mushroom (*Lentinus edodes*) not only as a food source but has been used as a medicine in China for hundreds of years. It is known to have an anti-carcinogenic action as well as positive effects on the immune system. The mushrooms come in a variety of forms including dried, fresh, extracts, and pills. Fresh mushrooms can be added to other foods and eaten daily, or a tea can be concocted by boiling 10 grams of mushrooms with 4 cups of water and then allowing the mixture to steep for 5 to 10 minutes. The tea should be ingested three times daily.

Reishi mushroom (*Ganoderma lucidium*) is related to the shitake mushroom and has also been utilized in China for medicinal purposes for a lengthy period of time. It has also been known to have a positive effect on the immune system. While fresh reishi mushrooms can be obtained or grown, it is more likely that they will be found in a dry or powdered form, which can be concocted into a tea and taken three times daily, as with the shitake.

Green leafy vegetables such as Chinese broccoli, Chinese kale, and bok choy are best blended with equal amounts of celery and parsley. Initially, 3 ounces mixed with equal amounts of water (and honey if desired) should be taken twice daily and then 8 ounces taken twice daily thereafter.

Royal jelly, produced from the salivary glands of worker bees as food for the queen bee, is available in liquid and tablet form. Reported to have excellent restorative properties it should be ingested daily. Sea cucumber is also felt to have restorative properties and can be ingested in salads or as a vegetable daily. Beef and pork liver, both high in iron, should be taken at least twice weekly.

Effective Chinese Herbs

Radix codonopsitis • *Dang shen*
This dried root of the *Campanulaceae* family is said to replenish qi and promote calmness between the spleen and stomach.

Radix angelicae sinesis • Angelica • *Dang gui*
Traditionally believed to nourish and supplement. Pharmacologically, is shown to increase the metabolic rate.

Rhizoma atractylodis • Atractylodes • *Bai zhu*
Traditionally said to aid qi while creating harmony in the spleen. Pharmacologically, acts to promote use of blood sugars.

Typical Herbal Formula

Gui pi tang, composed of the following:
Rhizoma atractyloidis (Bai zhu) 10 g.
Radix angelica sinesis (Dang gui) 10 g.
Radix codonopsis (Dang shen) 12 g.
Radix glycyrrhizae (Gan cao) 5 g.

Radix astragali (Huang qi) 20 g.
Longanae arillus (Long yan rou) 15 g.
Radix saussureae (Mu xiang) 3 g.
Zizyphi spinosi semen (Suan zao ren) 15 g.
Radix polygalae (Yuan zhi) 6 g.

Anxiety

DEFINITION   Anxiety is a nervous disorder characterized by feelings of fear, restlessness, and nervousness, and of impending negative events. In laymen's terms, it is "the jitters." Anxiety is one of today's most frequently encountered emotional disorders and is generally treated with mild anti-anxiety medications such as tranquilizers, which may have secondary side effects.

SYMPTOMS   Myriad symptoms can accompany anxiety, ranging from very mild, as the anxiety one may feel after drinking too much coffee, to severe and debilitating nervousness which can prevent functioning. The most frequent symptoms are fidgeting, uncontrolled anger, insomnia, crying, inability to concentrate or complete tasks, feelings of impending doom, depression, panic, rapid heartbeat, mild to severe sudden sweating, sudden trembling and dizziness. These may be accompanied by other emotional symptoms such as depression. Anxiety can be a disorder unto its own or a symptom of other disorders, both physical and mental. Symptoms of anxiety usually have a sudden onset and usually occur when the individual is under stress or upset from a particular event or happening. While the natural tendency is to attempt to ameliorate the symptoms immediately by ingestion of beverages such as alcohol or soothing teas, these substances frequently enhance the symptoms. In some instances, severe anxiety attacks can mimic heart attacks. In any case, when there is chest pain it is prudent that one first rule out the possibility of a heart disturbance by seeking examination by a physician.

Foods high in carbohydrates aid the body in relaxation by raising the blood-sugar level. You might notice that after eating a heavy meal of pasta or potatoes, you feel suddenly tired. This is the effect of the blood-sugar level being raised by the carbohydrates that have been ingested. Foods high in oils have the opposite effect and therefore should be avoided. Persons who suffer from anxiety should pay attention to their diets, as some foods may exacerbate anxiety episodes. For instance, it is not infrequent that people who drink coffee in excess find themselves anxious and unable to concentrate.

A rice porridge or gruel is common fare in all areas of China. This nourishing porridge is high in carbohydrates and can be made by adding a cup of shortgrain rice to a quart of water. The mixture should be brought to a boil and then simmered slowly, stirring frequently until the rice is broken down and a thick soup is formed. More water can be added to the desired thickness. This can be easily cooked in a rice cooker or crock pot. One half hour prior to the completion of the cooking, a slice of ginger can be added for taste.

Ginseng is reported to have a stabilizing effect on the blood pressure while also having a stimulating effect on those who feel depressed and debilitated, symptoms frequently accompanying anxiety. Ginseng can be obtained in a variety of forms including teabags, capsules, powdered, or blended with other ingredients. For those who suffer from anxiety, it is recommended that ginseng not be taken in this latter form, as some of the other substances might enhance the anxiety.

Ginseng tea can be made by adding one teabag to 2 cups of boiling water and allowing the tea to steep for 5 minutes. One cup should be taken twice daily initially and increased to 3 to 4 cups per day. Ginseng can also be made into a soup. In this instance, 5 grams should be added to a quart of water. Bring to a boil and allow to simmer for 10 to 15 minutes before ingesting. In either of the above formulas, avoid taking ginseng 4 to 6 hours prior to bedtime.

Drinks and foods high in vitamin C protect the body from stress. Although vitamin C can be taken in tablet form, fresh juices high in vitamin C are preferable and recommended to be taken on a daily basis.

A vitamin C cocktail can be made by mixing equal amounts of oranges and carrots and extracting the juices. Taking 8 ounces twice daily is recommended. Although many teas may in fact exacerbate anxiety, chamomile tea is reported to relieve anxiety and to have a relaxing effect. This tea can be made by mixing 2 to 3 teaspoons of chamomile per cup of boiling water and allowing to steep for 8 to 10 minutes.

The herb valerian (*Valeriana officinalis*), reduces anxiety, particularly anxiety associated with insomnia. Available as a tincture and also in dried form, it makes an effective tea when 1 teaspoon of the dried herb is combined with 2 cups of boiling water and allowed to stand until cool (at least 1 hour). The mixture is then strained and a cup is taken three times daily. This mixture can be made in advance and kept in the refrigerator.

Kava (*Piper methysticum*), a type of pepper plant, has long been used medicinally for treatment of anxiety. In this country it is available primarily as an extract and is taken in doses of 40 milligrams three times daily. I do not recommend taking it in conjunction with other herbs or foods and suggest that if valerian does not have a positive effect after three to four weeks, kava be tried.

EFFECTIVE CHINESE HERBS

Radix ginseng • Ginseng • *Ren shen*
Traditionally used to supplement qi while removing bad qi; believed to soothe the soul and aid the spirit. Pharmacologically, it stimulates the nervous system and the adrenal gland.

Fructus jujubae • Jujube • *Da zao*
Traditionally said to bring harmony and peace to the spirit while aiding the spleen and stomach. Pharmacologically, has an anti-ulcerative effect.

Arteriosclerosis

DEFINITION   A condition in which the walls of the blood vessels, arteriole walls, become laden with deposits which thereby lessen the effectiveness of the blood vessels and render them susceptible to other disease processes. In layman's terms, arteriosclerosis is called "hardening of the arteries," which in fact well describes the end result of the laying down of products on the vessel walls. Because of their coating, the walls become brittle and lose their elasticity. Through auscultation, one may even hear the resulting abnormal sounds caused by the blood moving through constricted, coated walls.

SYMPTOMS   Symptoms of arteriosclerosis are evident relative to the decline in function of the organs whose blood supply has been compromised. If the blood vessels to the heart are sclerotic, the person has reduced blood flow to the heart muscle and is subject to angina, cardiac failure, infarction, etc. If the blood flow to the carotid arteries that carry blood to the brain are compromised, brain functioning is decreased. The health risks to sufferers of arteriosclerosis are great.

NATURAL FOOD REMEDIES

Those who suffer from arteriosclerosis must attribute their malady in part to dietary habits. As such, changes are necessary: the diet should be restricted in animal fats. In their place, the diet should be enhanced with mung beans, soybeans, and fish. Fish oils have proved to have a tonic effect and should included in the diet at least four times per week. Those who respond poorly to stress, who do not exercise, and who have a hereditary history of arteriosclerosis, must make every effort to alter those patterns over which they have some control.

Fish can be steamed with ginger and soybeans. Any fresh white-fish can be placed in a steamer and topped with ginger, garlic, and soybeans, both for flavoring and their nutritional value. Ginger, garlic, and soybeans all have therapeutic effects in helping to reduce arteriosclerosis and should be included in the daily diet in any form convenient.

Mung beans and soybeans can be ingested in a dry roasted form as a snack. Eating cooked portions daily will enhance the diet as well. Soybean lecithin is reported to aid in the reduction in arteriosclerotic deposits. Two tablespoons of lecithin can be taken daily. Hawthorn fruit is also reported to have a similar effect of reducing arteriosclerotic deposits. Extracts of the hawthorn berry are available, with 10 drops per day an effective dose.

Seaweed and kelp can be utilized in broth to create healthful soups. To each quart of water, greens of bok choy, Napa cabbage, and parsley should be added along with dried seaweed and kelp. Simmered for 10 to 15 minutes, the broth is extremely healthful.

Ginko, utilized in Oriental medicine for centuries, has been recommended for increasing blood flow and increasing vascular efficiency. One tablet of 40 milligrams taken twice per day is the usual dosage. Ginseng tea can be made by steeping a bag of ginseng in 2 cups of water for 5 minutes. It should be taken at least twice daily.

Juices of greens should be taken daily. One can be concocted by adding equal amounts of celery, parsley, and carrots. At least 8 ounces should be taken daily.

Grapefruit fiber has been found to be an effective aid in the treatment of arteriosclerosis. It can be added to the diet in the form of marmalade or can be candied. As a marmalade, the skins of grapefruit are covered with water and the mixture brought to a boil. The water is discarded, and the skins once again are covered with water and the mixture brought to a boil. The water is then discarded a second time. The peel is sliced thin and then boiled with the juice of an orange to which has been added two cups of sugar. Water may be added to aid in dissolving the sugar. The mixture is slowly simmered until soft; watch carefully to see that it does not burn.

EFFECTIVE CHINESE HERBS

Glycine sojae semen • Soybean • *Hei dou*
Traditionally believed to correct any deficiencies of the blood. Pharmacologically, aids in the reduction in deposits of cholesterol.

Ginkgo semen • Ginkgo • *Yin xing*
Traditionally used to strengthen qi. Pharmacologically, increases blood flow.

Radix angelicae sinesis (Dang gui) 9 g.
Rhizoma cnidii (Chuan xiong) 6 g.
Radix glycyrrhizae (Gan cao) 6 g.
Lumbricus (Di long) 6 g.
Commiphora myrrha (Mo yao) 6 g.
Carthami flos (Hong hua) 9 g.
Cyperi rhizoma (Xiang fu zi) 3 g.
Persicae semen (Tao ren) 9 g.
Gentianae macrophyllae radix (Qin jiao) 3 g.
Notopterygii rhizoma (Jiang huo) 3 g.

Arthritis

DEFINITION Also known as chronic multiple degenerative joint disease, more often simply arthritis, it is caused by the erosion of the cartilage lining the joint surfaces. This erosion can be from many causes, including the natural aging process, or chronic stress on a particular joint as from sports, injury, obesity, and others.

SYMPTOMS Pain in the joints when used, with feelings of stiffness. Symptoms may be most acute during changes in temperature, such as the onset of winter or wet weather, when using the joint, or upon rising in the morning. There may be some swelling or a feeling of heat in the affected area.

NATURAL FOOD REMEDIES

Willow (Salix spp.) is known as the origin of aspirin. Infuse 2 teaspoons of the bark in 2 cups of boiling water and allow to steep for several hours. Drink three times daily.

Chaparral (*Larrea divaricata*), commonly known as the creosote plant, has provided relief to sufferers of arthritis, and is available raw and in tablets. The natural herb is preferable and can easily be made into a tea by boiling 1 tablespoon in 1 quart of water, and allowing to steep at least 15 minutes. Take at least 8 ounces three times a day. Flavored with lemon or lime and sugar. As you experience positive benefits, increase the herb to 2 tablespoons per quart of water.

The desert plant yucca is also reported to provide relief from arthritis. While the plant is not readily available, it is available in tablet form. Take 1 tablet twice daily for the first week, then increase to 3 tables three times daily.

Fruit juices are especially helpful, particularly fresh cherry juice. Take 8 ounces twice daily. Garlic as well is beneficial for arthritis, particularly when joints become inflamed. While available in tablets, 2 to 3 raw cloves, crushed with honey and taken three times daily, is preferable.

Eliminating meats and other proteins from the diet is reported to relieve pain and swelling. It is suggested that meats be replaced with beans, grains, and soybean products.

EFFECTIVE CHINESE HERBS

Radix pulsatillae • Pasqueflower • *Bai tou wen*
Traditionally used to cool action of the blood and expel heat. Pharmacologically, dilates blood vessels.

Erythrinae cortex • Sea vine bark • *Hai dong pi*
Traditionally used to reduce swelling, move fluids, and relieve pain. Pharmacologically, it has an analgesic effect.

TYPICAL HERBAL FORMULA

Shen rong hu gu wan, consisting of:
Cornu cervi parvum (Lu rong) 2 g.
Radix ginseng (Ren shen) 5 g.
Herba ledebouriellae sesloidis (Fang feng) 33 g.

Radix aristolochae fangji (Fang ji) 25g.

Os tigris (Hu gu) 5 g.

Radix angelicae sinesis (Dang gui) 30 g.

Asthma

DEFINITION Asthma is characterized by paroxysmal constriction of the bronchi, causing the individual to experience severe difficulties in breathing along with characteristic wheezing, coughing, and a generalized feeling of an inability to inhale. An "attack," in layman's terms, occurs when the tubes which carry air to the distal portion of the lungs are in spasm. These tubes constrict or tighten and there is a reduced amount of oxygen that can be carried to the cells to be exposed to the blood. These attacks are recurrent and most commonly are brought upon by allergic reactions, or they may be brought upon by infection.

SYMPTOMS Persons who suffer asthma have spasmodic attacks with rapid breathing. Most know that they suffer from the disease, and therefore have some awareness when an attack is beginning. With the attack there is wheezing, anxiety, and a feeling of pressure on the chest with accumulation of phlegm and saliva and associated difficulty in expectorating. There is a characteristic heaving of the chest as the person attempts to get air into the lungs.

NATURAL FOOD REMEDIES

Ginger is known to have a positive effect in the treatment of asthma, and comes in a multitude of forms. The Chinese recommend fresh ginger, which can be taken as a tea. Simply place several slices of fresh ginger (it need not be peeled) in boiling water and allow the mixture to steep for 5 minutes. The liquid should then be sipped three times daily. This mixture may help relax anyone sensing a tightening in the chest. For those who do not particularly like the taste of ginger, it may help to add a teaspoon of honey.

Ginger can also be made into a very flavorful cold beverage. Simply place several tubers of ginger into a blender or food processor. Process the ginger until it is in a rough pulp form. Add a quart of boiling water, and sugar or honey to taste (usually 1 cup of sugar or 1 cup of honey). When the mixture has become tepid, add 1 tablespoon of yeast. Let the mixture sit in room temperature for an hour and then place in the refrigerator overnight. The next day, strain the mixture into a pitcher. The mixture will keep for up to 1 week refrigerated. Cold liquids can aggravate asthmatics; therefore, any liquid is best taken at room temperature or heated. Ginger can also be ingested in pill form, with 500 milligrams the usual daily dosage.

Pruni radicis cortex is the bark of the prunus tree and is effective as a tea in the treatment of asthmatic episodes, both as an active treatment or a preventative. The bark is placed in a quart of water, boiled for half an hour and then allowed to sit until the liquid is tepid. It is then strained and ingested as a tea.

Onion juice has a positive effect on bronchiole spasms. Simply blend the onions and ingest 2 ounces three times daily. To make the juice more palatable, mix with carrot juice or tomato juice and add spices to taste. It is not recommended that alcohol be added as alcohol has a counter therapeutic effect.

The herb *Tussilago farfara*, commonly known as coughwort, is used in India and Asia for relief of asthma and other bronchial disorders. The herb can be purchased in dried form and can be made into a tea by placing 1 ounce of the herb in 4 cups of water. The mixture is brought to a boil and then simmered for 5 minutes, allowed to cool and then strained. A cup of the tea should be ingested two to three times per day.

Garlic is now reported as being beneficial for asthma disorders. It is available in many forms but the Chinese recommend that it be taken fresh. Simply mince several cloves of garlic and add to soups, salads or other foods. Should you find the taste unacceptable, it can be taken in tablet form.

While not effective for all persons suffering from asthma, some who respond positively to the internal ingestion of aloe vera. To control and provide a regular dosage, the extract is recommended.

When the acute symptoms are in remission, a tea should be made by boiling 5 grams of bitter apricot seeds with 4 grams fresh ginger and red dates. This tea should be consumed twice daily. (CAUTION: bitter apricot seeds are toxic and should not be eaten in raw form.)

EFFECTIVE CHINESE HERBS

Belamcandae rhizoma • Blackberry lily • *She gan*
Traditionally believed to move through the lungs and dispel heat, removing swelling and toxins while expelling phlegm. Pharmacologically, it has a hypotensive effect while increasing amplitude of pulse.

Radix ephedrae • Ma huang
Traditionally said to move through the lung meridian and control diaphoresis and deficiency of qi. Pharmacologically, has a dilating effect on the blood vessels.

TYPICAL HERBAL FORMULAS

She gan ma huang tang, consisting of the following:
Belamcandae rhizoma (She gan) 5 g.
Rhizoma zingiberis recens (Sheng jiang) 5 g.
Rhizoma pinelliae (Ban xia) 5 g.
Radix epedrae (Ma huang) 5 g
Herba asari (Xi xin) 1 g.
Radix asteris (Zi wan) 5 g.
Flos farfarae (Kuan dong hua) 5 g.
Fructus jujubae (Da zao) 9 g.
Fructus shisandrae (Wu wei zi) 2 g.
      or
Radix glycyrrhizae (Gan cao) 5 g.
Herba epedrae (Ma huang) 5 g.
Fructus jujubae (Da zao) 8 g.
      or
Cortex cinnamomi (Gui pi) 5 g.
Radix paeoniae lactiflora (Chih shao) 7 g.
Radix astragali (Huang qi) 5 g.

Radix ledebouriellae (Fang feng) 5 g.
Rhizoma atractylodis (Bai zhu) 5 g.
Semen armeniacae amarcum (Xing ren) 5 g.
Radix glycyrrhizae (Gan cao) 1 g.
Cortex magnoliae officinalis (Hou pu) 1 g.

Bed Sores

DEFINITION Bed sores or stasis ulcers, also commonly known as pressure sores, are breakdowns in the surface tissue of the skin and underlying tissue due to pressure and disturbed circulation. This disorder usually occurs in the elderly, individuals confined to bed or chairs, or otherwise unable to move about. Circulation is restricted due to the pressure of their bodies at the areas in contact with the furniture surfaces. The resultant area of tissue breakdown is frequently a target for bacterial growth. The best treatment for bed sores is prevention by movement, proper diet, and keeping contact areas dry.

SYMPTOMS Erythematous (red) areas where the body is in contact with other surfaces, breakdown in skin tissue with resultant surface oozing, bleeding, tenderness, and pain. Untreated bed sores can be quite severe and if left untreated can even be life threatening.

NATURAL FOOD REMEDIES

Symphytum officinale, commonly known as comfrey, is a well known plant which grows in Asia and in other temperate areas. The roots of this plant have reported to have been particularly successful in the treatment of skin disorders secondary to stasis problems. The roots are cleaned, placed in a blender with a pint of water and pulverized. This mixture is then brought to a boil for 5 minutes. Another pint of boiling water is added and the liquid allowed to cool to room temperature. The solution can then be utilized as a cleanser for ulcerated areas. The roots of the plant can also be allowed to dry and then pulverized and added to Vaseline. This mixture is then applied to the ulcerated areas three times daily.

Callendula officinalis, commonly known as the marigold, is a well-known folk remedy for treatment of ulcerated skin disorders. To make a liquid mixture, place the petals of several plants in a blender with 6 ounces of distilled water. Blend and then bring the mixture along with another 6 ounces of water to a boil. Allow to simmer for 5 minutes and then strain the liquid into a sterilized bottle. This solution can be utilized as a cleansing liquid and can be combined with any soothing cream and applied to the wound two to three times daily.

Foods high in Vitamine C, such as fruit juices, should be taken daily in large doses. These foods aid in the healing of tissues. Equal amounts of parsley should be mixed with orange and carrot juices and 8 ounces should be taken daily. It is imperative that the above remedies be combined with a program of movement of the individual to relieve pressure on the infected areas as well with keeping those areas as dry as possible.

EFFECTIVE CHINESE HERBS

Ricini Semen • Caster Bean • *Bi ma zi*
Traditionally used to remove moisture and swelling as well as toxic elements. Pharmacologically causes lysis of red corpuscles. For external application.

Phellodendri cortes • Aloe • *Lu hui*
Traditionally used to remove heat while cooling the liver. Pharmacologically, has an anti-ulcerative effect. For external application.

Bladder Infections

DEFINITION An invasion of the urinary bladder, the sac which retains urine in the pelvic cavity, by pathogenic microorganisms and the resultant reaction of the tissues to these microorganisms. The causative factors for introduction of microorganisms into the bladder can be numerous, the most common being unsanitary practices that allow infected materials come into contact with the urethra opening.

SYMPTOMS The most common symptoms of this disorder are frequent and burning urination, pain in the lower abdomen, passing of urine which is cloudy and sometimes containing blood and pus, irritability, and low-grade fever. Bladder infections are more common in females than in males.

NATURAL FOOD REMEDIES

Arctostaphylos uva ursi, commonly known as uva ursi berry, is an evergreen plant that has been utilized in Asia for medicinal purposes. To concoct a tea, an ounce of the thick leaves are placed in 4 cups of water. The leaves are crushed and the mixture is brought to a boil, then allowed to steep until tepid. The crushed leaves are removed and a cup of tea is then taken three times daily. The uvi ursi berry tea has a diuretic action and has an antiseptic effect on the bladder tissues.

Cranberries also have an antiseptic effect on bladder tissue. The berries may be crushed and mixed with water which is then brought to a boil. The mixture is then allowed to cool and is strained, with 16 ounces of the liquid taken daily. Although cranberry drinks can be purchased, be aware that "cranberry cocktail" and cranberry juices mixed with other fruit juices may not contain sufficient cranberry to be effective.

Peppermint tea is also reported to have a beneficial effect. A tea can be made by pulverizing 0.5 ounce of peppermint leaves with 4 cups of boiling water and allowing it to cool. It should be taken three times daily. Strawberries have a similar positive effect. They can be ingested whole, with 6 ounces daily recommended, and also can be made into an herbal tea.

As much water as possible should be taken daily, up to 4 to 5 pints. To make the urine alkaline, a teaspoon of sodium bicarbonate should be added to each pint.

Phellodendri cortex • Phellodendron • *Huang bo*
Traditionally used to removes toxins, as it removes heat as well as fire. Pharmacologically, has an antibacterial and anti-inflammatory effect.

Ramulus cinnamomi • Cinnamon • *Gui zhi*
Traditionally used to promote the flow of qi while warming through the lung, heart, and bladder meridians. Pharmacologically, has an antibacterial and antiviral effect.

TYPICAL HERBAL FORMULA

Tong guan wan, consisting of the following:
Anemarrhenae rhizoma (Zhi mu) 25 g.
Ramulus cinnamomi (Gui zhi) 3 g.
Phellodendri cortex (Huang bo) 25 g.

Cancer

DEFINITION   Cancer or malignant disorders are a cellular growths or tumors whose growth is uncontrolled. Because of the uncontrolled growth, secondary tumors occur which invade the surrounding tissues and then extend to other areas of the body. There are many types of cancer.

The concept of cancer in Chinese medicine is entirely alien to that of Western medicine. To the Chinese physician, cancers typically have their origin in emotional disorders that create a block in the flow of energy, resulting in stagnancy in the tissues. The response of the body to overcome this stagnancy is abnormal or increased growth, hence tumors or accelerated growth of tissue forms. While disruption in the flow of energy and fluids within the body may have internal causes, such as the emotional disorders mentioned, disruption may also occur from external forces, such as toxic elements from industry that are released into the environment, food additives, etc.

The approaches to treatment of cancer by Western and Chinese physicians are consequently entirely different. While treatment in the West is centered on surgical procedures to remove or chemical agents to "kill" the cells of the cancerous growths, the Chinese method of treatment, primarily herbal, is centered on removing accumulation of fluids, restoring the normal flow of fluids and energy, and counteracting toxic elements. Even when Western methods are utilized in China, such as surgery or chemotherapy, herbal remedies are utilized to counteract the toxic effects of the chemotherapy and to normalize the flow of body fluids and energy.

Can herbal therapies cure cancer? Western physicians would claim that herbal remedies alone can not. Chinese physicians would claim the contrary. However, there is now evidence that chemical agents in some herbal remedies indeed do have anticarcinogenic properties, and when used in combination with other therapies contribute to an effective treatment regimen. Some herbs prove also to be effective in enhancing the immune systems.

NATURAL FOOD REMEDIES

Ganoderma lucidium, known in China as *ling zhi,* is a fungus that grows in mountainous, wooded areas. Utilized for centuries as a medicinal agent, it is said to have a positive effect on the immune system. The dried fungus is typically concocted into a tea or ingested in soups, and is available in a dried, powdered form.

Shiitake mushroom is reported to have an effect similar to the *ling zhi* fungus, and has also been utilized for medicinal purposes for centuries. Recent reports indicate that it may well aid in interferon production. Shiitake mushrooms are available raw or dried and also in tablets.

Garlic is also reported to have immune enhancing properties. Those who take it regularly are reported to have decreased incidence of carcinoma of the gastro-intestinal areas.

Oldenlandiae herba • Oldenlandia • *Bai hua she she cao*
Traditionally used to remove stagnancy and toxins. Pharmacologically, has an antibacterial effect and in cultures has been shown to reducethe growth of cancer cells.

Radix subprostratae sophorae • Sophora subprostrata •*Shan dou gen*
Traditionally used to disperse fluids and toxins. Pharmacologically, has an anticancer effect in animal studies.

Scutellariae barbatae herba • Scutellaria • *Ban zhi lian*
Traditionally used to disperse fluids and toxins. Pharmacologically, has a bacteriostatic effect on abnormal leukocytes.

Zedoariae rhizoma • Zedoaria • *E shu*
Traditionally used to disperse fluids and toxins as well as mobilize qi. Pharmacologically, has an anticancer effect in laboratory tests.

Wedeliae herba • Wedelia • *Ma lan jin*
Traditionally used to disperse swelling and fluids while removing toxins. Pharmacologically, has an anticancer effect in laboratory tests.

Radix wikstroemiae • Wikstroemia • *Pu yin gen*
Traditionally used to disperse fluids and toxins. Pharmacologically, has a carcinostatic effect in laboratory tests for cervical carcinoma and lymphadenoma.

Violae herba • Viola • *Zi hua ti ting*
Traditionally used to remove toxins and heat. Pharmacologically, has an antibacterial effect.

Shark cartilage is said to inhibit the growth of blood vessels in cancerous growths; as the blood vessels are unable to supply nutriments to the growths, the growths in turn are reported to shrink. Although large-scale studies have not rendered conclusive evidence, many cases have been reported in which cancerous tubers have disappeared. Shark cartilage can be obtained in herbal pharmacies and taken in tablet form.

Canker Sores

DEFINITION   Technically known as *aphthous stomatitis*, canker sores are small, circular mouth ulcers that are usually white or yellow and surrounded by a red raised area that is tender and painful. They usually have a sudden onset and appear on the mucous membranes of the lips, mouth, and gums and are extremely painful. Pain is somewhat related to the fact that while eating or talking, the sores rub against the tongue or adjacent tissues. These sores are believed to be viral in origin and related to stress or irritating foods.

SYMPTOMS   The most common symptom is sudden pain with a circular round mouth ulcer appearing on the gum, tongue, or mucous membrane of the mouth. They usually appear suddenly and as single sores.

NATURAL FOOD REMEDIES

A soothing tea can be made of rosemary and myrrh which is effective in washing the area and promoting healing. A tablespoon of dried rosemary or, preferably, a sprig of fresh rosemary is lightly crushed in a cup to which has been added 10 milliliters of tincture of myrrh and 2 cups of boiling water. The mixture should be allowed to steep 5 minutes and then sipped at moderate temperature, taking care to allow the fluid to bathe the canker sores, at least three times daily. When one feels a canker sore coming, this remedy should be instituted immediately. Clove oil, which for some has a healing effect, can be applied directly to the ulcer.

Avoid liquids that are either extremely hot or extremely cold and also avoid eating foods which are highly irritating such as nuts and other rough grains. Vitamin C and beta-carotene-rich foods promote healing. A drink of leafy green vegetables such as Chinese broccoli, bok choy, and carrots can be mixed with equal amounts of orange juice, with 8 ounces taken daily.

An effective mouthwash can be made utilizing the herb red sage, which has an anti-inflammatory action. Simply add a tablespoon of the dried herb to a quart of boiling water in a sterilized jar. I like to add zest of lemon also. Allow to cool and strain. If you are one who suffers from canker sores, try this as a daily mouthwash.

It is known that people prone to canker sores are more apt to suffer from them during periods of stress. A stressful lifestyle with a diet high in caffeine, fats, and alcohol only enhances the possibility of creating internal stress for your body.

EFFECTIVE CHINESE HERBS

Commiphora myrrha • Myrrh • *Mo yao*
Traditionally used to promote the movement of stagnant blood and healing. Pharmacologically, has a soothing effect while being antifungal.

Carbuncles

DEFINITION   Commonly called boils, carbuncles are infections of the skin usually due to a *staphylococcus* bacteria. The lesion typically is round, with a raised red border and a large, draining, pus-filled center. The lesion and surrounding area is usually extremely painful and hot to the touch. Carbuncles usually appear as single disorders of the skin, although some people are prone to repeated episodes.

SYMPTOMS   A round, red lesion with an indurated border, raised and painful. The center seeps pus and serous fluid.

NATURAL FOOD REMEDIES

Echinacea angustifolia, commonly known as the coneflower, is effective in the treatment of carbuncles. Tincture of echinacea is readily available; 2 drops can be mixed with a juice and taken every two to three hours. It can also mixed with distilled tepid water in the same ratio and applied to the carbuncle four times daily. I particularly recommend bathing of the carbuncle with this liquid as it not only promotes healing but cleanses the infected area. Handle all dressings carefully and change frequently.

Comfey can also be made into an effective bathing liquid, mixing 4 ounces with 2 cups of boiling water and allowing the mixture to steep as it returns to room temperature. Bathe the carbuncle four times daily.

Juices rich in vitamin C also promote healing. A particularly effective mixture can be made of equal amounts of beets, carrots, and parsley or Chinese broccoli, with 8 ounces of the liquid taken daily.

EFFECTIVE CHINESE HERBS

Radix echinopsis • Rhaponticum and echinops • *Lou lu*
Traditionally used to remove toxins and pus while dispelling heat. Pharmacologically, has an anti-inflammatory effect.

Siegesbeckiae Herba • St. Paul's wort • *Xij jian cao*
Traditionally used to reduce surface infections while dispelling wind. Pharmacologically, has an antibacterial effect.

Cold and Cough

DEFINITION   The common cold is an illness caused by a virus, usually characterized by a group of symptoms associated with mild upper respiratory distress. Colds are frequent, annoying, and easily spread from one person to another. Colds usually occur with changes of the seasons in spring and winter and should be heeded, as they can progress to more serious respiratory diseases if the immune system of the body is sufficiently weakened.

SYMPTOMS   Colds exhibit a group of symptoms usually including cough, mild fever, nasal obstruction and discharge, watery eyes, sore throat, and a general feeling of mild malaise.

I highly recommend taking juices rich in vitamin C on a regular basis, not only after one has become ill. Vitamin C promotes healing, and there is documentation supporting the fact that those who take large amounts of vitamin C have less frequent colds and other ailments. Grapefruit juice, freshly squeezed, is the most beneficial of the citrus juices, with 8 ounces taken daily.

Leafy green vegetables with a high beta carotene content are also effective. A particularly effective drink can be made from mixing equal amounts of bok choy, parsley, and Chinese broccoli, taking 6 ounces daily for the first day and every day thereafter until symptoms disappear.

Licorice root has an antiviral property and is particularly effective when combined with astragalus, long used in Chinese medicine. Try making a tea by steeping a tablespoon of the dried root in 2 cups of boiling water. Add a half teaspoon of tincture of licorice root and take a cup three times a day. It not only has healing properties but it also promotes perspiration.

Garlic is reported to be effective in the treatment of colds. While it is available in a variety of forms, one can simply ingest several cloves of garlic that have been crushed and mixed with honey. This same mixture can be allowed to steep in a cup of boiling water and then sipped. It is especially soothing to the throat. Echinacea is also effective for severe congestion and throat irritation. Available in tincture form, 10 drops should be added to 8 ounces of fruit juice and taken four times daily.

For a tea effective in soothing a painful cough, try combining 1 teaspoon each of licorice, aniseed, and hyssop in 4 cups of boiling water. Add some honey and sip it warm. Another remedy is made of 1 tablespoon of hyssop tincture alone mixed thoroughly with a cup of honey. Keep it in the refrigerator, and during coughing episodes, take a half teaspoon. Besides being soothing, the hyssop has both antispasmodic and anti-inflammatory actions.

When your nose aches from chronic blowing and you feel your nasal passages are stuffed, try adding moisture to the air by vaporizing. Ever notice how much better you feel in the kitchen? Try adding moisture to your environment by using a vaporizer or by sitting in your kitchen while a large pot of water simmers on your stove. Add a tablespoon of chamomile flowers and marjoram to the boiling water.

Allii fistulosi bulbus • Chinese chive • *Cong bai*
Traditionally used to promote yang, aiding blood circulation and diaphoresis. Pharmacologically, has an antibacterial effect as well as an antipyretic effect.

Thymi serpylli herba • Thyme • *Di jiao*
Traditionally said to have a warming action to disperse cold. Pharmacologically, has a protective action on the bronchi.

Radix glycyrrhizae • Licorice • *Gan cao*
Traditionally used as a toxin remover, bringing qi to a harmonious level while removing heat. Pharmacologically, has anti-inflammatory, antispasmodic, and detoxifying effects.

TYPICAL HERBAL FORMULA

Herba schizonepetae (Jing jie) 10 g.
Radix peucedani (Qian hu) 10 g.
Radix platycodi (Jie geng) 9 g.
Radix notopterygii (Jiang huo) 10 g.

Constipation

DEFINITION Constipation is usually a misunderstood disorder. Technically it is a lessening of the frequency of bowel movements or defecation; a retention of feces. However, the frequency is dependent upon the habits of the particular individual. For some individuals, daily bowel movements are the norm; for others, once every other day is the norm. Disruption of the normal bowel pattern is usually a symptom of other disturbances, such as a change in dietary habits, a lack of exercise, a reduction in fluid intake, emotional disturbance, etc. Causative factors of constipation are innumerable, ranging in severity from intestinal obstruction due to a growth in the intestine, volvulus (a twisting of the intestine causing an obstruction), to a lack of food intake, to lesser severe ailments such as influenza, stress, or alteration of sleep patterns. While constipation is usually not a serious disorder, in some instances it can be quite severe.

SYMPTOMS In general, constipation accompanied by vomiting, fever, and abdominal pain requires greater intervention than constipation resulting from minor ailments such as colds and influenza or the simple effects of travel. The herbal remedies recommended here are for minor ailments or alterations in the usual bowel patterns of the individual, either a decrease in frequency of defecation or of dry and hard feces.

NATURAL FOOD REMEDIES

Tackle your constipation in a systematic manner. Increase the moisture to your bowel, increase the bulk in your food, and stimulate your bowel with natural herbal products.

Dandelion root increases moisture going to the bowel, while bulk can be increased by high-fiber vegetables and grains, and cascara *(Rhammus purshiana)* can add a mild stimulation. Dandelion root and cascara can be concocted by combining a teaspoon of dandelion root and a teaspoon of cascara in 2 cups of boiling water. Allow to cool to room temperature and sip before bedtime.

Leafy green vegetables such as bok choy, Chinese kale, gaai laan, and Chinese chives can be ingested in a variety of forms, although for this particular disorder, it is recommended that the whole vegetables be eaten to increase the fiber content. A salad of bok choy mixed with Chinese chives is particularly effective.

Licorice, available in extract form, is effective. Mix 8 to 10 drops of the extract with 8 ounces of water and a tablespoon of honey and lemon. Ginseng is also effective, particularly as a tea taken three times daily. When teabags are available, simply place a bag in a cup of boiling water and allow the brew to steep for at least 5 minutes. White fungus can be made into a mild soup. Combine 4 ounces with 6 cups of water, bring the mixture to a boil, and allow to simmer for 10 minutes. A cup should be taken twice daily. Children find fresh water chestnuts tasty and they are effective treatment. Peel the chestnuts and place them in a mixture of honey and the juice of one lemon. Slice thinly and ingest. Apricots and oranges can be mixed with the water chestnuts for an effective fruit combination. Coffee also has a natural laxative effect. Simply drink a cup of coffee each morning.

EFFECTIVE CHINESE HERBS

Ruta graveolens • Rue • *Da huang* (family)
Traditionally used to clear away internal heat and bring moisture internally. Pharmacologically, has an antibacterial effect and is also felt to be anti-carcinogenic.

Fructus forsythia • Forsythia • *Lian qiao*
Traditionally used to clear internal heat as well as toxins. Pharmacologically, has an antiviral, antibacterial effect.

Aurantii fructus immaturus • Bitter orange • *Zhi shi*
Traditionally used to encourages qi circulation. Pharmacologically, stimulates gastrointestinal function.

TYPICAL HERBAL FORMULA

Rhei rhizoma (Da huang) 4 g.
Radix phiopogonis (Mai men dong) 5 g.
Natrium sulfuricum (Mang xiao, Pu xiao) 5 g.
Rehmanniae radix (Sheng di huang) 14 g.
Radix scrophulariae (Xuan shen) 7 g.

Depression

DEFINITION An emotional condition characterized by feelings of dejection, loss of hope, and melancholia, in layman's terms, "the blues." Depression can vary from feeling mildly down to a point where one may feel totally immobilized and suicidal. Therefore, it is important that if one's feelings begin to approach any thought of self destruction or if the depression does not dissipate after a short period of treatment, it is important that a physician be consulted. Depression can be a normal feeling that follows a traumatic event such as the loss of a loved one, loss of a pet, or loss of a job; however, after a relatively short period of time, the depressed feeling should begin to dissipate. These remedies may help shorten the period of depression and also may aid those persons who are prone to mild depressions or blue feelings, including those which normally accompany medical conditions such as painful menstruation.

SYMPTOMS Loss of appetite, feelings of helplessness, lack of involvement, withdrawn behavior, crying spells, insomnia, remaining in bed and sleeping excessively, weakness, and, in severe cases, thoughts of self-destruction.

NATURAL FOOD REMEDIES

St. John's wort has recently been the subject of so many news reports as being effective in the treating of depression. This "newly discovered" herb has, in fact, been utilized for getting rid of the blues for hundreds of years, but only recently is being looked at seriously after several research studies have indicated positive evidence of its ability to alleviate depression. As well, it is being studied for its potential to suppress H.I.V. production. St. John's wort is so called because it flowers around June 24th, the birthday of St. John the Baptist, while wort is Old English for plant. Now available in a variety of forms, a tea can be made by steeping 1 teaspoon of the herb in a cup of boiling water for 10 minutes. It is then strained and taken three times daily. In the alcohol extract form, an eighth of a teaspoon is mixed with fruit juice and taken three times daily. It is important to keep in mind that effects are not immediate; one or two weeks may be needed before its positive effects are felt. Those who may experience mild gastrointestinal disturbance should take it with meals. Do not combine this herbal remedy with any medication unless your physician is informed and advises you of the suitability of the treatment. There are also reports that people who take St. John's wort on a regular basis may be sensitive to sunlight.

Sage is also known to reduce depressed feelings. Mix 1 tablespoon of sage in 2 cups of boiling water and allow to steep. Strain and then mix with honey. A tea can also be made with fresh sage leaves, which is preferable. In this instance, take several fresh leaves and crush with a spoon, add boiling water, and allow to steep. Add sweetener to taste and ingest twice daily. Passion flower is frequently combined with sage and is available in a tincture form. Simply add 10 drops of the tincture to each cup of sage or honey tea.

Liquorice tea as well can aid in the reduction of depressive symptoms. Extract of liquorice can be added to water to form a tea which is flavored with honey. This should be taken three to four times daily.

Evaluate your diet. Processed foods, foods with caffeine and alcohol, and foods with high sugar content may contribute to depressed feelings and should be eliminated from the diet. A high-fiber diet and a diet which is high in proteins should be instituted.

Effective Chinese Herbs

Curcumae tuber • Tumeric • *Yu jin*
Traditionally used to promote the flow of qi and dissolve stagnant qi. Pharmacologically, stimulates heart and breathing.

Radix scutellariae • Scute • *Huang qin*
Traditionally used to remove toxins and moisture. Pharmacologically, has a tranquilizing effect.

Rhizoma atractylodis • Atractylodes • *Bai zhu*
Traditionally used to create peace in the stomach and spleen while toning qi through the stomach meridian. Pharmacologically, has a diuretic and sedative effect.

Radix bupleuri (Chai hu) 8 g.
Radix paeoniae alba (Bai shao) 8 g.
Cyperi rhizoma (Xiang fu zi) 8 g.
Aurantii fructus (Zhi ko) 8 g.
Rhizoma cnidii (Chuan xiong) 8 g,
Radix glycyrrhizae (Gan cao) 6 g.
Rhizoma atractylodis (Bai zhu) 8 g.

Diarrhea

DEFINITION Diarrhea is a condition in which there are frequent abnormally watery fecal discharges. It usually has a sudden onset and frequently is associated with some other ailment such as eating overly spiced or improperly cooked foods, drinking non-potable water, other dietary factors, a viral or bacterial infection, metabolic disease, stress, etc.

Diarrhea not associated with a sudden onset due to an accompanying disorder, or containing blood in the stool, or long lasting may well be a symptom of a more serious underlying disorder of the bowel and should be investigated by a physician immediately. Any diarrhea which does not respond to treatment within a relatively short period of time warrants immediate attention.

SYMPTOMS A disruption of the normal excretory pattern of the individual, resulting in watery and frequent stool, usually accompanied by associated gastric distress, loss of appetite, nausea, general feelings of malaise, and sometimes fever. Diarrhea can be a symptom of many ailments, such as cold, influenza, overeating, irritation by various foods, or one symptom of more serious ailments such as partial bowel obstruction, liver disease, parasite infection, etc. The herbal remedies here are treatment of diarrhea secondary to minor infections such as a cold or influenza and gastric distress secondary to a dietary problem.

Because diarrhea expels large amounts of water from the body, it is important that any remedy include the ingestion of large amounts of fluid. Along with fluid loss is loss of many minerals, which, therefore, should be included in the fluid intake.

Lemon balm (*Melissa officinalis*) and cranesbill (*Geranium maculatum*) are two herbs which combine to make an effective treatment. Both have an anti-inflammatory action. Simply combine 1 teaspoon of each with 2 cups of boiling water and allow to steep for 10 minutes. Drink throughout the day until your symptoms subside, particularly after you have had a diarrhea episode.

Ginger is therapeutic in the treatment of diarrhea. Simply crush several slices of ginger and add 8 ounces of hot water. Allow to steep for 5 minutes, then add 1 tablespoon of honey, 1 teaspoon of baking soda, and a pinch of salt. This mixture should be taken at least four times daily.

Apples contain pectin, which aids in the treatment of diarrhea. Simply blend cored apples with honey to taste and take at least four times per day. Carob powder, itself is a successful treatment, can be added to the apple mixture or any fruit juice.

Pepper can be mixed in the ratio of 1 to 9 with sugar, ground into a powder, and then mixed with water. One tenth of the mixture should be ingested three times per day in 8 ounces of liquid; take daily until the symptoms disappear. If the mixture is not to your taste, mix with honey and lemon juice.

Blackberry tea made from the leaves of the blackberry bush can be taken three to four times daily. Simply crush the leaves or steep 1 teaspoon of the herb in a cup of boiling water, adding honey to taste. This tea is made from the leaves of the plant and should not be confused with blackberry flavored teas, which are totally unrelated.

Rice gruel is an old Chinese treatment. This common breakfast food should be taken three times a day as long as symptoms persist. For children or adults who do not relish the taste, simply mix in a blender with a banana and a teaspoon each of vanilla and honey. The banana will replenish lost minerals lost and provide bulk. The apple mixture mentioned above can also be added to the gruel for a change of taste.

Aloe • Phellodendri cortex • *Lu hui*
Traditionally used to reduce internal heat, kill fungus and intestinal parasites, and relieve constipation. Pharmacologically, has a purgative effect and is reported to be anti-carcinogenic.

Coix lacryma jobi • Job's tears • *Ma yuen* (variation)
Traditionally used as a detoxicant, a diuretic, and to dispel heat. Pharmacologically, acts as a diuretic.

Allii bulbus • Garlic • *Da suan*
Traditionally used to control diarrhea while removing dampness. Pharmacologically, is antispasmodic and anticancerous.

TYPICAL HERBAL FORMULA

Herba agastachis (Huo xiang) 9 g.
Radix platycodi (Jie geng) 2 g.
Folium perilae (Zi su zi) 9 g.

Diminished Sexual Desire

DEFINITION Loss of desire for sexual intercourse may have various causes, including pressure from work, emotional loss, or some underlying sexual conflict or problem in your relationship. However, there are also instances of hormone deficiencies or disturbances such as depression. The following remedies are no substitute for resolving conflicts with your partner, or solving external problems.

SYMPTOMS Loss of sexual desire, loss of sexual interest, and general lack of desire for intercourse. Usually a symptom of a primary disturbance such as stress, emotional difficulties with the partner, depression, disturbance of ego perception. However, when a lack of sexual desire accompanies one of these conditions, the person is usually aware of it.

Ginseng is reported to be beneficial in the treatment of lack of sexual desire. Available in a variety of forms, Korean ginseng is preferable and should be taken three to four times daily in the tea form.

Increasing dopamines will aid in awakening sexual desire. Soybeans are particularly effective for this and should be taken daily. Cooked soybeans are preferable, and one should not expect to have the beneficial effects by ingesting products such as soy sauce. Fava beans are also rich in dopamine and can be added to the daily diet. Excessive fat and sugar intake should be curbed.

Pulsatilla, while not said to increase sexual desire in an of itself, does aid in increasing aggressiveness. Available in a tincture form, 5 centiliters can be added to tepid liquids and taken three times per day.

EFFECTIVE CHINESE HERBS

Radix pulsatillae • Pulsatilla • *Bai tou wen*
Traditionally used to cool the blood. Pharmacologically, it dilates the peripheral blood vessels.

Diverticulitis

DEFINITION The pouches of the colon, diverticulum, become irritated by food trapped in them. The intestine becomes inflamed and infected, and in serious cases can mimic the signs of a bowel obstruction.

SYMPTOMS Abdominal pain and cramping, which usually follows eating items that become obstructed in the diverticulum, such as seeds, nuts, corn, etc. This disorder, once detected, usually reoccurs. Other symptoms can include fever, nausea, vomiting, blood and mucus in the stool, and general malaise.

One of the most important treatments lies in restricting the diet once symptoms have appeared. Seeds, nuts, grains, nuts, and foods with high roughage content should be elimanated from the diet; these hard items can get caught in the pouches of the intestine.

To relieve the intestine of gas, a tea can be made by mixing charcoal with tepid water and sweetened with honey and lemon. This should be taken four times daily.

Fenugreek (*Trigonella foenum graecum*) has an extensive history of use for medicinal purposes. An effective tea in the treatment of diverticulitis is made by mixing 1 teaspoon of fenugreek seeds per cup of boiling water. After steeping 5 minutes, the liquid is strained of the seeds and taken three times per day.

A juice high in beta carotene should be taken daily to enhance healing. Equal amounts of spinach, Chinese kale, bok choy, and Chinese broccoli should be extracted of their juices, with 8 ounces ingested daily.

Effective Chinese Herbs

Trigonellae semen • Fenugreek • *Hu lu pa*
Traditionally used to remove cold and warm the yang. Pharmacologically, it acts to reduce mucus.

Dysmenorrhea

DEFINITION   Painful menorrhea, in layman's terms, painful periods or PMS, premenstrual syndrome. Menstruation is controlled by the hormones estrogen and progesterone. Therefore, when these hormones are in excess or lacking, different symptoms arise.

SYMPTOMS   Dysmenorrhea is usually characterized by a variety of symptoms, which may include swelling, water retention, tenderness in the breasts, pain in the lower abdomen, back and sacral area, heavy menorrhea, irritability, depression, and general feeling of malaise.

At the first sign of swelling, switching to a complete vegetarian diet, low in fat, is recommended. Proteins are not only hard for the body to digest but they also are more apt to make the body retain water during menorrhea. A vegetarian diet aids diuresis which will reduce swelling in the body.

Raspberry leaf (*Rubus spp.*) is both high in minerals and also aids the female body of menstrual cramps. Make a tea from the leaves of the raspberry with a tablespoon of the dried herb in a cup of boiling water. Allow to steep and then strain and add sweetener if desired.

Korean ginseng taken three times daily reduces pain and promotes metabolism. Available in teabags or powdered, it is easily prepared by steeping in water. To promote circulation, add fresh spearmint leaves to boiling water along with sliced fresh ginger and allow to steep for 5 minutes. Sweeten to taste and take three times daily. Cinnamon tea also reduces menstrual distress. Bark of cinnamon can be steeped in boiling water, 1 stick per 2 cups. Add ginger to the mixture to help reduce swelling.

Celery root and lotus root cooked in equal amounts and ingested daily is helpful for irregular menstruation. Equal amounts of celery and fennel juice are effective in that both are high in phytoestrogens. Add 6 ounces of this juice to cooled ginseng tea and take at least twice daily.

Rhizoma cnidii • Cnidium • *Chuan xiong*
Traditionally used to promote blood circulation and fortify qi. Pharmacologically, has an antispasmodic effect while also being a vasodilator.

Radix paeoniae alba • White peony • *Bai shao*
Traditionally used for menorrhagia to supplement blood. Pharmacologically, has an antispasmodic effect.

Cyperi rhizoma • Cyperus • *Xiang fu zi*
Traditionally used to regulate menses and aid functioning of the liver. Pharmacologically, inhibits muscle spasm.

Rhizoma corydalis tuber • Corydalis • *Yan hu suo*
Traditionally used to promote flow of qi and blood circulation. Pharmacologically, acts to relax muscles.

TYPICAL HERBAL FORMULA

Rhizoma cnidii (Chuan xiong) 5 g.
Radix angelica sinensis (Dang gui) 5 g.
Radix paeoniae alba (Bai shao) 5 g.
Persicae semen (Tao ren) 5 g.
Carthami flos (Hong hua) 5 g.
Auranthii fructus (Zhi ko) 6 g.
Rhizoma corydalis tuber (Yan hu suo) 5 g.

Edema

DEFINITION   The presence of above normal amounts of fluid in the interstitial tissues of the body, seen as swelling most commonly visible in the extremities. Causative factors are wide ranging, including cardiac failure, liver disease, and retention of fluids secondary to hormonal change in the menstrual cycle.

SYMPTOMS   Puffiness in the face, eyelids, and lower limbs, discharge of scant amounts of urine, congestion in the chest, and a heavy feeling in the body.

NATURAL FOOD REMEDIES

The following herbal remedies are designed to promote the flow of water in the body. Bring 30 to 40 grams of Job's tears and 2 cups of water to a boil. Allow to steep for 5 minutes, strain, and add brown sugar to taste. Drink as a tea at least twice daily.

Slice the peel of a grapefruit into slivers and boil in 2 cups of water. Add 1.5 cups of sugar and simmer until the peel is soft. Remove the peel, roll it in sugar, and let dry. Keep in an airtight jar and take regularly.

Soak red beans and cook with garlic and ginger until very soft. Eat one cup daily.

Make a broth using 4 large cloves of garlic, onion, grated ginger (1 to 2 slices), and a bit of parsley and chives in 1 cup of water. Do not add salt. Simmer until garlic is soft and ingest.

EFFECTIVE CHINESE HERBS

Phaseoli semen • Red bean • *Chi xiao dou*
Traditionally used as a diuretic, to remove swelling, and to remove heat. Pharmacologically, has a diuretic action.

Arecae pericarpium • Areca peel • *Da fu pi*
Traditionally used to cause movement of water, reduce swelling, and move qi to descend. Pharmacologically, has a diuretic action.

Zanthoxyli bungeani semen • Zanthoxylum • *Jiao mu*
Traditionally used as a diuretic, to remove abdominal water. Pharmacologically, has a diuretic action.

Radix phytolaccae • Poke root • *Shang lu*
Traditionally used as a purgative, and to expel water, thereby causing a reduction in swelling. Pharmacologically, has a diuretic action.

TYPICAL HERBAL FORMULA

Shu zao yin zi, consisting of:
Rhizoma alismatis (Zi xie) 5 g.
Areca semen (Bing lang) 5 g.
Phaseoli semen (Chi xiao dou) 8 g.
Rhizoma seu radix notoptergii (Jiang huo) 5 g.
Arecae pericarpium (Da fu pi) 5 g.
Poria cocos (Fu ling) 5 g.

Radix phytolaccae (Shang lu) 5 g.
Zingiberis exocarpium (Jiang pi) 8 g.
Zanthoxyli semen (Jiao mu) 5 g.
Gentianae macrophyllae radix (Qin jiao) 5 g.
Aristolochiae caulis (Mu dong) 5 g.

Emphysema

DEFINITION Emphysema is a serious disorder of the lungs whereby there is air in the connective tissues caused by rupture of the pulmonary alveoli. In layman's terms, the air sacs in the lungs burst from chronic irritation and the air enters the spaces in the surrounding tissues. Obviously, the ability of the lungs to function effectively is sorely compromised. Emphysema is condition commonly seen in persons who experience chronic lung irritation, such as long-term smokers and those working in heavily polluted areas such as coal mines. Although non-reversible, every effort must be made to prevent its progression and to treat the existing symptoms.

SYMPTOMS Dyspnea or shortness of breath, cough, a heaving chest, weakness, loss of weight, a general feeling of debilitation, cough, rapid pulse, and aversion to wind and cold. The chest cavity also is seen to be rigid and expanded.

NATURAL FOOD REMEDIES

First and foremost, the progression of the disease must be stopped. Therefore, the first step is to remove the irritant. If it is a pollutant, the pollutant must be removed. Smoking or any exposure to smoke must be terminated at once.

The small shrub rhubarb has been used for medicinal purposes for lung disorders for centuries. It is now known that its leaves contain ephedrine, which is beneficial in lung disorders because it causes shrinkage of mucus membrane tissue. Available through herbalists, it can be taken in trial doses of 3 grams daily.

Licorice is available in as tincture and can be combined with crushed ginger to form an effective tea. Crush several slices of ginger and add to boiling water. Allow to steep for 5 minutes and then add the tincture of licorice. This mixture should be sipped when tepid at least four times daily.

Ginseng also provides relief from coughing episodes. It should be taken four times daily. Both coffee and tea are stimulants and can be taken up to four times daily to provide some relief from labored breathing.

The most effective treatment for this disorder likely requires a combination of herbs. I have found a particularly effective tonic or treatment can be made of rhubarb, licorice, hawthorn, elecampane, and wild cherry bark. Combine 1 teaspoon of each of these herbs as tinctures and take once daily. It can be also be mixed with carrot juice or grapefruit juice. After a week, increase to three times a day.

Effective Chinese Herbs

Poria cocos • Hoelen • *Fu ling*
Traditionally said to eliminate dampness and while soothing the mind warms the middle. Pharmacologically, has both tranquilizing and diuretic effects.

Fructus schizandrae • Schizandra • *Wu wei zi*
Traditionally said to clear the lungs while drying. Pharmacologically, has a stimulating effect on the central nervous system while also being an antitussive.

Radix asteris • Aster • *Zi wan*
Traditionally thought to enter through the lung meridian, breaking up phlegm and relieving cough. Pharmacologically, has a diuretic effect as well as an ability to cause expectoration.

Radix ginseng • Ginseng • *Ren shen*
Traditionally thought to enter through the lung meridian, supplementing yin and qi while expelling bad qi. Pharmacologically, is cardiotonic and stimulating to the central nervous system and the adrenal gland.

Eriobotryae folium • Loquat • *Pi pa ye*

Traditionally used to cleanse lungs and move qi. Pharmacologically, is an antitussive while stimulating the respiratory center of the central nervous system.

TYPICAL HERBAL FORMULA

Eriobotryae folium (Pi pa ye) 10 g.
Radix ginseng (Ren shen) 5 g.
Radix astragali (Huang qi) 10 g.
Mori cortex (Sang bai pi) 10 g.
Radix ophiopogonis (Mai men dong) 10 g.
Radix rehmanniae praeparata (Shou di huang) 10 g.
Radix asteris (Zi wan) 10 g.

Enhancing the Immune System

DEFINITION   The human body has its own extraodinary defense mechanism, the immune system. It consists of a complex group of distinctive cells, each of which plays a specific role. These cells include the lymphocytes, the main cells of the system, and those cells which interact with the lymphocytes, the monocyte/macrophages, dendrite cells, langerhans cells, natural-killer cells, mast cells, and others. There are two classes of lymphocytes, B lymphocytes, which are the precursors of antibody secreting cells, and T lymphocytes, which impart regulatory functions such as helping or inhibiting an immune response, lysis of virus-infected cells or certain neoplastic cells.

A simplistic view of the workings of the system is as follows: When an invading organism is found in the system by T cells, the T cells assault the organisms chemically. They also attract macrophages, which digest the invaders. When B cells find the invaders, they produce antibodies which neutralize or destroy them. To counter the production of T and B cells, so that they do not become invasive to the body itself, there are suppressor cells to keep cell ratios of in check. However, if for some reason suppressor cells are in excess, the immune functions of the body can be suppressed, which makes the body vulnerable to invading viruses and bacteria.

NATURAL FOODS TO ENHANCE THE IMMUNE SYSTEM

Shiitake mushrooms have long been utilized in Chinese medicine. They are available dried and also fresh and can be readily added to the diet. The common garlic plant has among its many properties an ability to enhance the immune system. Simply supplement your daily diet with garlic cloves three times daily.

There are many types of ginseng, but Siberian ginseng in particular is reported to have immune enhancing properties. Now available in a variety of forms, it can be taken three times daily as prescribed; however, it is most easily taken as a tea three times daily.

Aid your immune system by taking control of your diet. Reduce your meat and cholesterol intake while increasing your intake of fibers, leafy green vegetables, and fruits. This is a more natural, Oriental diet in which meat intake is much less than in the West.

CHINESE HERBS FOR ENHANCING THE IMMUNE SYSTEM

Radix astragali • Astragalus • *Huang qi*
Traditionally said to suppliment qi while dispersing water. Pharmacologically, has a cardiotonic and a tonifying effect as well as a diuretic effect. Aids in T cell production.

Carthami flos • Carthamus • *Hong hua*
Traditionally used to dispel stagnant blood and enhance circulation. Pharmacologically, dilates the coronary arteries to vitalize the blood.

Curcumae tuber • Tumeric • *Yu jin*
Traditionally said to dissolve qi stagnation. Pharmacologically, has a stimulating effect.

Ganoderma • Lucid ganoderma • *Ling zhi*
Traditionally said to disperse accumulation while tonifying. Pharmacologically, has an antihepatic effect, reducing symptoms of hepatitis.

Radix ginseng • Ginseng • *Ren shen*
Traditionally supplements qi. Pharmacologically is said to tonify and stimulate DNA production.

Radix codonopsitis • Codonopsitis • *Dang shen*
Traditionally said to replenish qi. Pharmacologically, stimulates the nervous system and increases body resistance.

Ophiopogonis tuber • Ophiopogon • *Mai men dong*
Traditionally said to moisten, cleanse, and remove heat. Pharmacologically, has a toning effect and anti-inflammatory effect.

Gallbladder Disease

DEFINITION   The gallbladder is a gourd-shaped organ located on the underside of the liver that functions as a reservoir for bile. When diseased, it commonly develops an inflammation sometimes accompanied by gall stones, both of which inhibit the flow of bile. As bile is associated with the emulsification and absorption of fats in the intestine, when the gallbladder is diseased, these functions are disturbed as well.

SYMPTOMS   The most common symptom associated with gallbladder disease is abdominal pain and discomfort, usually following a fatty meal. This pain is usually in the mid-epigastric area of the abdomen and is accompanied by nausea, tenderness when deeply palpated, loss of appetite, belching, bad breath, foul-smelling yellowish stools, and vomiting. It is not uncommon to experience pain in the shoulder blades or in the right shoulder. Usually the person suffering from this disease, statistically more likely to be an overweight woman, is aware that the symptoms usually follow ingestion of a oily meal.

The diet of a person suffering with gallbladder disease should be restricted in fats and increased in fibers and fruits. Soybeans and red soybeans are particularly nourishing and aid in the reduction of cholesterol. Both can be made into soups as well as mixed with leafy green vegetables; red soybeans are commonly ingested at the end of a meal as a dessert. While the gallbladder is in distress, the diet should include red soybeans at least once daily. Tumeric, used for gallbladder disease in Chinese medicine, is available as a powder. A teaspoon can be added to the beans or soup.

Fruits, particularly those with pectin, have found to have some effect in dissolving gallstones. Peppermint, also, contains oils which aid in the dissolving of gallstones. The leaves of 2 tablespoons of the dried herb should be infused with 5 cups of boiling water, steeped for 5 minutes, and taken two to three times per day.

Celadine, either the plant or extract, is highly effective. Add 8 to 12 drops of the extract to orange juice or carrot juice and take twice daily. Spinach and parsley can be blended in equal amounts and then combined with an equal amount of carrot juice, with 8 ounces taken daily.

A natural Chinese remedy is to boil banana peels and corn silk in a quart of water for 15 minutes. The mixture is then strained and 8 ounces of the liquid ingested daily.

Crataegi fructus • Hawthorn • *Shan zha*
Traditionally used to improve the digestion of food and remove food stasis. Pharmacologically, crataegolic acid increases gastric secretions thereby aiding in the digestive process.

Massa medicata fermentata • Medicinal leaven • *Shen gu*
Traditionally used to move qi and enhance digestion. Pharmacologically, improves digestion by the presence of amylase and yeast.

Bao he wan, consisting of:
Crataegi fructus (Shan zha) 10 g.
Massa medicata fermentata (Shen gu) 10 g.
Raphanus sativus (Lai fu zi) 10 g.
Fu ling (Poria cocos) 10 g.
Citrus tangerina (Zhu pi) 3 g.
Rhizoma pinelliae (Ban xia) 10 g.
Fructus forsythiae (Lian qiao) 10 g.

Gingivitis

DEFINITION Gingivitis is an infection of the gums that can progress to more serious pyorrhea. It is a disease which warrants treatment by a dentist, as it is a progressive disorder which can result in loss of teeth and severe mouth infections. Gingivitis usually begins with deposits of tarter along the gum lines. Tarter harbors bacteria and the gums subsequently become infected. The treatments listed here are both preventative and therapeutic, and suggested to be used in conjunction with treatments by your dentist after consultation with him or her.

SYMPTOMS Soreness and redness of the gums, accompanied by bad breath, oozing about the gum line, and ultimately, fever, chills, loosening and loss of teeth.

NATURAL HERBAL REMEDIES

Both myrrh and echinacea have found to have antibacterial effects. They are available as tinctures and can be easily combined by place two drops of each with your toothpaste when brushing after meals. To cleanse the infected area, add the tincture to warm water, wash the infected areas at least three times a day and before bedtime.

Although aniseed does not have an antibacterial effect, it does have the pleasant taste and odor of anise and can be utilized to freshen the breath. Combine several drops of the tincture with warm water and rinse several times during the day. Chamomile also has a pleasant odor and taste and can be utilized as a mouthwash. Prepare a cup of chamomile tea but allow it to cool and use it as a mouthwash instead of drinking it.

I personally like a mixture of dried peppermint leaves, a gentle stimulant, combined with equal amounts with dried hibiscus flowers in 2 cups of boiling water. Allow to cool to room temperature, add three drops of echinacea, and use as a mouthwash and rinse.

TYPICAL HERBAL FORMULA

Huang lian shang qin wan pian, consisting of:
Rhei rhizoma (Da huang)
Chrysanthemi flos (Ju hua)
Coptidis rhizoma (Huang lian)
Fructus gardeniae jasminoidis (Shan zhi zi)
Rhizoma ligustici wallichi (Chuang xiong)
Herba schizonepetae (Jing jie)
Radix ledebouriellae (Fang feng)
Radix scutellariae (Huang qin)
Radix platycodonis grandiflori (Jie geng)
Gypsum *(Shi gao)*
Radix angelicae sinesis (Bai zhi)
Radix glycyrrhizae uralensis (Gan cao)
Fructus viticis (Ma jing zi)
Fructus forsythiae (Liang qiao)
Flos inulae (Xuan fu hua)
Phellodendri cortex (Huang bai)
Menthae herba (Bo he)

This mixture comes prepared in tablet form.

Gout

DEFINITION Gout is a disorder caused by the deposit of uric acid in the joints of the body. Uric acid is a natural product formed in the breakdown of cells; however, when there is excess in the bloodstream and more than can be excreted, the uric acid seeps into joint tissues causing pain and swelling. This disorder is more often seen in men than women, more often found in those who suffer from obesity, and more often found in persons who suffer from arteriosclerosis and high blood pressure. There is also a familial pattern in some cases.

SYMPTOMS Pain and swelling in the joints, particularly those of the lower extremity, and the large toes.

NATURAL FOOD REMEDIES

Persons who suffer from this disorder must reevaluate their diets. Meats should be excluded, particularly organ meats such as liver, brains, kidneys, and the like. Intake of vegetables, grains, and fruits should be increased. Alcohol intake should be curtailed and water intake should be increased to at least eight 8-ounce glasses per day. Rapid weight loss should be avoided.

Cherry and celery juice have proven effective in the treatment of gout. Extracted from the fresh fruit or vegetable, 8 ounces of the juice should be taken daily.

Common parsley is a strong diuretic, with the leaves, stems, and roots all effective. Parsley can be pulverized in equal amounts with celery, the juices extracted, and 8 ounces taken twice daily. Parsley can also be taken as a tea by infusing the leaves and roots with boiling water and taken four times daily. Simply crush a large bunch of parsley and roots, add 4 cups of boiling water and a tablespoon of celery seed, and allow to steep 10 minutes. As there is stimulation of smooth muscle, pregnant females should not take this remedy.

Willow *(Salix spp.)* is known as the original source of aspirin. Two tablespoons of the bark infused with 2 cups of boiling water and allowed to stand until cool should be taken three times daily. This mixture can be made in large quantities and stored in the refrigerator.

Ribwort (*Plantago lanceolata*) is a common plant in Asia and Europe but not in America. The dried plant is effective in promoting the excretion of excess uric acid. You can dry the plant itself or you can purchase the dried leaves, with the usual dosage 2 grams per day. If you purchase the dried leaves and roots, simply crush 1 tablespoon in two cups of boiling water and allow to steep for at least a half hour. Ingest a cup three times per day.

Effective Chinese Herbs

Desmodii herba • *Jin qian cao*
Traditionally used to eliminate dampness while clearing damp heat. Pharmacologically, promotes diuresis.

Hangover

DEFINITION   Hangover is the common name for the feeling that one has the day after overindulging in alcoholic beverages. It is really a disturbance in the electrolytes caused by overindulgence. While not a serious disorder, it can be quite distressful for those suffering from it.

SYMPTOMS   May include throbbing headache, hypersensitivity to noise, light, and emotions, feelings of nausea, mild stomach upset, diarrhea, and general malaise.

Natural Food Remedies

The most remarkable recent addition to the many traditional hangover cures is kudzu. This plant was imported from Japan to control erosion along highways and has become known as the "weed of the

South" because of its rapid growth of almost several inches per hour. Thought a useless and destructive plant at first, it was discovered to be useful as a soup thickener, like cornstarch, and now is believed to have a remarkable effect in treatment of drinking problems (see *Alcohol Abuse*). It not only reduces the intensity of that "morning after" feeling but seems to reduce the desire for excessive alcohol intake. Make a tea of the kudzu plant by drying the roots and leaves after cleaning them, and steeping overnight about an inch of the dried root with some crushed leaves in 4 to 6 cups of boiling water. Take a cup of this tea before retiring. If you do not like the taste, add a squeeze of lemon juice and a teaspoon of honey. Before retiring, drink at least 12 ounces of water.

Foods high in sodium help rehydrate the body. Salted soybeans, foods to which soy has been added, salted Chinese mustard greens, and preserved fish are all helpful in aiding retention of fluids.

A mixture of juices high in vitamin C such as orange, grapefruit, or strawberry aids in rehydrating the body while providing vitamin C that helps remove alcohol from the body. Of all of the citrus juices, grapefruit is the most beneficial.

A mixture of carrots, Chinese broccoli, celery, beets, and parsley in equal amounts should be pulverized and the juices extracted, with 8 ounces of the mixture taken prior to sleep.

Nux vomica, long used in Chinese herbal medicine, is now available in tablet form. One tablet can be taken upon arising along with fluid to help rehydrate.

EFFECTIVE CHINESE HERBS

Strychni semen • Nux vomica • *Ma qian zi*
Traditionally used to eliminate swelling upon entering through the liver and spleen meridians. Pharmacologically, has the effect of promoting blood circulation while stimulating the central nervous system, and increasing activity of the stomach and intestine.

Hay Fever

DEFINITION More technically known as allergic rhinitus, this is a disorder of the upper respiratory system. As the causative factor is usually pollens, the ailment is seasonal in occurrence. Although treated in the West primarily with medications, the secondary effects of some medications are equally troubling.

SYMPTOMS Common symptoms of allergic rhinitis are sneezing, running nose with clear fluid, cough, tearing, nasal congestion, and general malaise.

NATURAL FOOD REMEDIES

Red onions are effective, taken in raw form or in a tincture. When taken in the latter form, 30 milliliters taken twice daily is an effective dose. An interesting drink can be made by pulverizing red onion and celery, extracting the juice and then adding an equal amount of carrot or tomato juice. At least 8 ounces should be taken twice daily during the height of hay fever season. Carrot juice, 6 ounces twice daily, also relieves symptoms.

One tablespoon of cebadilla seeds steeped in a cup of boiling water for 5 minutes and then ingested as a tea is highly effective, as are Job's tears, with 5 grams steeped in 2 cups of boiling water for 5 minutes and taken in two equal doses daily.

Coltsfoot (*Tussilago farfara*) is particularly effective in the relief of coughing and sneezing. A tea can be made with 1 tablespoon in 4 cups of boiling water. Allow to steep for 10 minutes, strain, and drink 1 cup twice daily.

EFFECTIVE CHINESE HERBS

Radix astragali • Astragalus • *Huang qi*
Traditionally used to reduce swelling, release water, increase yang, and promote qi. Pharmacologically, has diuretic, antiviral, and vasodilative effects.

Rhizoma atractylodis • Atractylodes • *Bai zhu*
Traditionally used to reduce dampness, release water, and aid qi.
Pharmacologically, has diuretic and sedative effects.

TYPICAL HERBAL FORMULA

Yu ping feng san, consisting of:
Rhizoma atractylodis (Bai zhu) 8 g.
Radix astragali (Huang qi) 20 g.
Radix ledebouriellae (Fang feng) 8 g.

Headache

DEFINITION Headache generally refers to pain is experienced anywhere in
the head area. Excluding headaches from trauma, this disorder is
usually seen as a symptom of an underlying disorder whose etiology
can be wide ranging, with tension, emotional trauma, or changes in
temperature or hormone balance the most frequent causes. Headaches can be also caused by growths within the cranium. In most
cases, these headaches are accompanied by neurologic disturbances;
any persistent headache should be evaluated thoroughly by a doctor.

SYMPTOMS A sensation of drumming, compressive, or stabbing pains in
the head, any of which can be accompanied by anxiety, irritability,
fearfulness, disturbance in eating, and vomiting. Migraine
headaches, a particular type of headache characterized by an aura
or symptom preceding the headache, are frequently accompanied
by a sensation of flashing lights, nausea, and acute pain in the head
made more severe by light.

NATURAL FOOD REMEDIES

People may respond quite differently to the natural food remedies
for headaches. However, in general headache sufferers would ben-

efit from restricting intake of food additives, caffeine, and tannin, and increasing their water intake. Fresh ginger and primrose oil should be added to at least one meal daily. They should learn to relax, or at least be aware of and avoid causes of tenseness, such as loud noises and bright lights. And, of course, smoking should be stopped and alcohol intake reduced.

Effective treatments include juices rich in coumarins, which have provided relief from migraine headaches. Equal amounts of celery, carrot, and cucumber juices should be combined, with 8 ounces taken twice daily.

Several dried or fresh leaves of feverfew, fresh preferably, should be steeped in 2 cups of boiling water, crushing the leaves against the side of the cup with a spoon. Add a teaspoon of honey and sip when tepid twice daily. This aid is not recommended for pregnant females or children below age five.

Rosemary, peppermint, marjoram, lavender, or thyme can all be made into effective teas. In each case, a teaspoon of the dried herb can be added to 1 cup of boiling water, allowed to infuse for 5 minutes and then sweetened with honey. Do not initially combine any of the herbs, but take separately to find which is effective in your own case.

Agnus castus is particularly effective for headaches related to menstrual difficulties and swelling. Available in tablet form, it should be taken twice daily.

The herb "self heal" (*Prunella vulagaris*) relieves tension and has a hypotensive effect. It can be infused by mixing 5 grams with 2 cups of boiling water. The usual dosage is 3 cups per day.

Effective Chinese Herbs

Corydalis tuber • *Yan hu suo*
Traditionally used to reduce qi stagnation and blood stasis. Pharmacologically, promotes blood circulation and relaxes smooth muscle

Menthae herba • Mentha • *Bo he*
Traditionally used to disperse wind and heat. Pharmacologically, is a blood dilator with analgesic and antipruitic effects.

Rhizoma cnidii • Cnidium • *Chuan xiong*
Traditionally used to move qi and dispel wind. Pharmacologically, has an antispasmodic effect while also being a vasodilator.

Radix ledebouriellae • Siler • *Fang feng*
Traditionally used to reduce dampness and wind. Pharmacologically, has an antipyretic effect.

Strychni semen • Nux vomica • *Ma qian zi*
Traditionally used to reduce pain and swelling. Pharmacologically, stimulates the central nervous system.

TYPICAL HERBAL FORMULA

Menthae herba (Bo he) 3 g.
Rhizoma cnidii (Chuan xiong) 9 g.
Angelicae radix sinesis (Bai zhu) 6 g.
Ledebouriellae radix (Fang feng) 6 g.
Radix glycyrrhizae radix (Gan cao) 6 g.
Rhizoma seu radix (Jiang huo) 6 g.
Herba schizonepetae (Jing jie) 9 g.

Heartburn

DEFINITION Also known as acid reflux, a burning sensation in the esophagus that follows a meal of spicy, greasy, or heavy foods late in the evening, caused by stomach acids backing up into the esophagus. Persons who experience heartburn frequently have repetitive episodes. One should note that heartburn can mask cardiac symptoms; however, with heartburn one does not have difficulty in breathing or swallowing, dizziness, or bloody or black stools. If any of these symptoms are present, one should seek medical attention.

SYMPTOMS A burning sensation which usually follows overeating or eating highly spicy foods. The discomfort usually occurs when one has gone to be and is in the reclining position or when wearing tight clothing. Obese people are more likely to suffer from this disorder.

NATURAL FOOD REMEDIES

Evaluate your diet. Avoid fatty, oily, or highly spiced foods late in the evening; in fact, do not take any food for three hours before retiring. In place of fatty, high-calorie foods, one should eat high-fiber foods such as beans, grains, and fruits. A cup of soup made of red soybeans settles the stomach at the end of a heavy meal.

Tea made by steeping slices of ginger in boiling water and allowed to steep for 10 minutes should be sipped after heavy meals. A tea can also be made by crushing star anise and steeping it with 2 cups of boiling water for 5 minutes. The mixture is then strained and ingested slowly. The star anise and ginger teas can be mixed.

Make a therapeutic tea of comfrey root and chamomile. Make a tea of comfrey root by steeping 1 teaspoon of the herb in 2 cups of boiling water, then adding it to two cups of your chamomile tea. Take 1 cup at least three times a day, sipping after each meal.

EFFECTIVE CHINESE HERBS

Rhizoma zingiberis recens • Fresh ginger • *Sheng jiang*
Traditionally thought to move through the lung, spleen, and stomach meridians, to warm, control vomiting, and remove toxic substances. Pharmacologically, stimulates the action of the stomach and has an antiemetic effect.

Heart Disease

DEFINITION Coronary heart disease is a disturbance of occlusion or partial occlusion of the coronary artery vessels. This is a particularly severe ailment, as the coronary artery vessels carry blood to the walls of the heart and thereby supply nutriments to the heart muscle.

With a reduction in food supply to the heart muscle, its function is compromised. If there is total occlusion of one of the blood vessel, the heart wall is deprived of nutriments and therefore cannot function; this is life threatening.

SYMPTOMS   When the coronary heart vessels are occluded, symptoms include dyspnea, or difficulty in breathing, shortening of breath, lightheadedness, pressure on the chest that feels like squeezing and may intermittently be relieved and then reappear, radiating pain to the neck and arms, perspiration, palpitations, and sometimes a feeling of impending doom. When such symptoms appear, immediate medical treatment is warranted.

NATURAL FOOD REMEDIES

Evaluate your diet. While hereditary factors and emotional temperament are important, medical studies show that diet has a remarkable relationship to coronary heart disease. Intake of red meats, dairy products, and processed foods should be replaced with grains, fruits, fresh vegetables, fish, and skinless chicken.

Soybean lecithin, available in liquid form, is reported to aid in the reduction of occlusion of blood-vessel walls and in the reduction of blood cholesterol. It is recommended that 2 to 4 tablespoons of lecithin be taken three times daily. Yellow soybeans can be cooked until soft, with 1 cup taken daily.

Hawthorn (*Crataegus oxycantha*) has been utilized for medicinal purposes in a long time. It is reported to have positive effects in the reduction of arteriosclerotic deposits. Extract of hawthorn is available, with 10 to 15 drops taken three times daily.

Molasses and honey have been used in the treatment of cardiac disease. Between 2 and 4 tablespoons of honey should be mixed with hot water and taken three time daily. Molasses is high in B complex vitamins; an effective tea can be made by adding 1 teaspoon per cup of boiling water and ingested twice daily.

Lightly cooked or raw leafy green vegetables high in beta carotenes, such as Chinese broccoli and kale, should be taken as least once daily.

Ginkgo semen • Ginkgo • *Yin xing*
Traditionally believed to aid qi. Pharmacologically, is antibacterial, reduces cholesterol, and dilates blood vessels.

Rhizoma pinelliae • Pinellia • *Ban xia*
Traditionally used to enter through the spleen and stomach meridians to disperse accumulation and swelling while removing dampness. Pharmacologically, has a sedative effect.

Bulbus allii chinensis • Chinese chive • *Xie bai*
Traditionally used to promote yang and the flow of qi in the chest. Pharmacologically, reacts on the smooth muscle.

TYPICAL HERBAL FORMULA

Gua lou xie bai ban xia tang, composed of:
Rhizoma pinelliae (Ban xia) 15 g.
Bulbus allii macrostemi (Xie bai) 18 g.
Trichosanthis fructus (Gua lou) 15 g.

Heat Rash

DEFINITION Heat rash, commonly known as "prickly heat," is a skin condition caused by failure of the sweat glands to exude sweat through the pores; the sweat literally gets trapped in the skin. While not itself a severe disorder, it is an indication that the overheated body is failing to exude sufficient sweat, and if chronic, medical attention should be sought.

SYMPTOMS A bright red rash which appears after exercise or exertion, with feeling like someone is sticking pins into the skin.

Aloe can be crushed and the creamy liquid applied lightly to the affected area twice daily. Guava also provides relief. Simply pulverize the fruit and apply the liquid to a soft towel. Hold the towel against the affected areas for 30 minutes three times daily.

In spite of the fact that one afflicted will feel overheated, do not apply ice to the erythematous areas. Rather apply cool water for 30 minutes, pat dry and then apply aloe for 30 minutes and repeat.

Green leafy vegetables should be ingested immediately and continued until there is relief. Chinese broccoli, mustard greens, and bok choy should be combined in equal amounts and the juices extracted. This should be combined with an equal amount of water and 8 ounces taken three times daily.

Effective Chinese Herbs

Cera flava • Beeswax • *Feng la*
Traditionally used to promote tissue regeneration while reliving pain and removing toxins. Pharmacologically, has a soothing, healing effect.

Solani herba • Nightshade • *Long kui*
Traditionally used to reduceswelling by dispelling heat and removing toxins. Pharmacologically, has anti inflammatory properties.

Hemorrhoids

DEFINITION Hemorrhoids are infections of the venous blood vessels of the rectum. Commonly called piles or rectal piles, one can suffer from both internal or external hemorrhoids. Most persons who suffer from hemorrhoids have repetitive episodes. Females who are pregnant frequently suffer from hemorrhoids due to the excess pressure on the anal blood vessels.

SYMPTOMS Symptoms for this disorder vary according to the severity of the infection. Most common are itching, protruding tissue extending from the anus, soreness of the rectal area, pain upon sitting and defecating. In severe cases there is rectal bleeding, thrombosis of the blood vessels in the anal area, extreme discomfort and pain, vomiting, nausea, fissures, constipation, emotional irritability, and fever.

NATURAL FOOD REMEDIES

The diet should be immediately changed to increase intake of fiber and fruits. Red soybeans and yellow beans can both be made into a highly nourishing and effective soup by simply boiling in water with garlic and ginger. Continue to add liquid while the beans are simmering until they are soft and the soup has a medium consistency. Take at least once daily.

The change in diet will also produce a softer stool. *Do not strain* when having bowel movements, but do not avoid bowel movements because they may be painful. Avoiding bowel movements will cause increased pressure on the rectal area, leading to further distress. Blackberry and cherry juice, 8 ounces twice daily, will provide vitamins and also soften the stool.

For treatment of painful extruding internal or external hemorrhoids or fissures, sit in the tub on a soft towel in a few inches of hot water, as hot as can be tolerated, and a cup of witchhazel. The towel allows greater exposure of the hot water to the painful area. Continue to add heated water to maintain the temperature for at least 20 minutes in order to accomplish a thorough soaking of the area. Pat dry and apply crushed aloe both internally into the rectum and the external area. Repeat at least four times daily while remaining off of the feet during the day.

Further relief can be obtained by making a strong mixture of black tea, allowing the tea to cool, and applying it with a compress to the rectal area three times daily.

Another topical ointment can be made by combining 30 grams of *Ranunculi ternati radix*, the Chinese herb *Mao zhua cao*, with 250 grams of sunflower oil and 25 grams of beeswax. Heat gradually until the material combines, let cool, and apply needed.

Cimfuga rhizoma (Sheng ma) 5 g.
Radix glycyrrhizae (Gan cao) 5 g.
Radix bupleuri (Chai hu) 5 g.
Rhei rhizoma (Da huang) 10 g.
Radix semiaquilegiae (Tian kui zi) 5 g.
Radix scutellariae (Huang qin) 10 g.

High Cholesterol

DEFINITION Cholesterol is a fatty alcohol substance which is present naturally in the body. An above normal level of cholesterol as well as a high level of LDL cholesterol relative to HDL cholesterol in the body substantially increases one's susceptibility to many diseases, including cardiac disease. When one has a high cholesterol, the excess fats in the blood begin to deposit plaques on the blood vessel walls, causing a loss of elasticity of the blood vessels. This reduces their effectiveness and increases the possibility of heart attack and strokes.

SYMPTOMS Weakness, loss of consciousness, swelling, chest pain or pressure with simple exertion, leg cramps, generalized discomfort in the legs with simple walking, malaise, above normal perspiration, joint pain, and chest congestion.

NATURAL FOOD REMEDIES

If you do not evaluate your diet and reduce your intake of fats, no remedy can be successful. Increase your intake of fish, fowl (with skin removed), fruits, vegetables, and high-fiber foods, while reducing to a minimum, or to none, your consumption of red meat.

Ginseng aids in the reduction of blood cholesterol. Simply infuse a ginseng teabag with boiling water, allow to steep for several minutes, ingesting at least three times daily. If you dislike the flavor, ground ginseng or pills are both available.

Garlic also aids in the reduction of blood cholesterol, and can easily be added to foods daily. Try crushing a clove of garlic and mixing it with a bit of honey or maple syrup. Or crush a clove of garlic with syrup and add wine vinegar for a gourmet salad dressing. It can also be taken in tablet form. A surprisingly palatable garlic tea can be made by steeping 6 cloves of garlic in cool water for 6 hours. Add chives or cinnamon to taste and have a cup three times daily.

Highly effective in reducing cholesterol, soybean lecithin is available as an oil. Simply use in place of your regular oil in making salad dressing. Both apples and carrots have a high pectin content and aid in removing cholesterol. Pulverize fresh carrots and apples to make a pleasing mixture, and drink 8 ounces twice daily.

Used in Chinese medicine for hundreds of years, ginkgo is now available in a variety of forms including tablets and extracts. Take three times daily.

EFFECTIVE CHINESE HERBS

Ginkgo semen • Ginkgo • *Yin xing*
Traditionally used to enhance qi. Pharmacologically, has an effect of reducing cholesterol.

Poria cocos • Hoelen • *Fu ling*
Traditionally used to harmonize the "middle warmer" while promoting diuresis. Pharmacologically, it has a nutritive effect as well as a diuretic effect.

Allii bulbus • Garlic • *Da suan*
Traditionally used to promote diuresis and diaphoresis. Pharmacologically, has an antihypertensive as well as an antibacterial effect.

TYPICAL HERBAL FORMULA

Xiao zhi tang, composed of:
Poria cocos (Fu ling) 12 g.

Nelumbinis folium (He ye) 12 g.
Chrysanthemi flos (Ju hua) 12 g.
Cassiae torae semen (Jue ming zi) 15 g.
Lonicerae caulis et folium (Ren dong teng) 15 g.
Coicis semen (Yi yi ren) 15 g.
Maydis stigmata (Yu mi xu) 10 g.
Alismatis rhizoma (Zi xie) 12 g.

Hypertension

DEFINITION   When one has a high blood pressure, the heart must work harder, placing increased pressure on blood vessels and increasing the risk of strokes. Causes of hypertension include essential (those without known cause), adrenal (caused by adrenal ischemia), portal (secondary to cirrhosis of the liver), and others. The herbal remedies listed are primarily directed towards essential, vascular, and benign hypertension.

SYMPTOMS   Headaches, vertigo, flushed face, insomnia, frequent loss of control of temper, poor response to stress, and in some cases swelling.

NATURAL FOOD REMEDIES

Blackstrap molasses has been used as a successful remedy for hypertension. It can be added to other liquids, such as herbal teas, and taken three times daily. One recipe calls for the juice of half a lemon, a teaspoon of blackstrap molasses, and 1 cup of boiling water.

Celery is utilized as an antihypertensive food, and can be taken in a variety of forms, three times daily. Pulverize the celery and extract the juices, drinking 6 ounces three times daily, or blend with carrot juice, in which case 8 ounces should be taken three times daily. A Chinese recipe includes dicing the celery and mixing with rice-wine vinegar. Cook until tender and eat three times daily.

Bring to a simmer a third of a cup of rice-wine vinegar combined with 6 grams of ginger and some sugar. Strain the juice and ingest twice daily.

Peel 4 to 5 fresh water chestnuts and add to the juice and peel of a mandarin orange. Boil with a cup of water and ingest as a tea.

EFFECTIVE CHINESE HERBS

Radix bupleuri • Bupleurum • *Chai hu*
Traditionally said to disperse heat and congestion, raise yang and promote qi. Pharmacologically, has both tranquilizing and antiphlogistic effects.

Radix scutellariae • Scute • *Huang qin*
Traditionally used to remove toxins, promote diuresis, dry moisture, remove heat, and quell fire. Pharmacologically, has both diuretic and hypotensive effects.

Radix angelicae sinesis • Angelica • *Dang gui*
Traditionally used to promote the movement of blood and relive excess moisture. Pharmacologically, has a diuretic effect and relaxes smooth muscles.

TYPICAL HERBAL FORMULA

Lang dan xie gan tang, consisting of:
Rhizoma alismatis (Ze xie) 9 g.
Rehmanniae radix (Sheng di huang) 15 g.
Radix bupleuri (Chai hu) 9 g.
Radix angelicae sinesis (Dang gui) 9 g.
Plantaginis semen (Che qian zi) 10 g.
Radix glycyrrhizae (Gan cao) 2 g.
Radix scutellariae (Huang qin) 10 g.
Gentianae radix (Long dan) 3 g.
Aristolochiae caulis (Mu dong) 12 g.
Fructus citrus tangerina (Zhi zi) 9 g.

Hypotension

DEFINITION Hypotension is an abnormally low blood pressure.

SYMPTOMS Characterized by dizziness upon arising, fatigue, coldness in the extremities, particularly in the hands and feet, a systolic blood pressure usually below 90 millimeters upon sitting or standing, fainting spells, palpitations, and feelings of anxiousness.

NATURAL FOOD REMEDIES

Ginger is reported to normalize blood pressure. An effective tea is made by adding several slices to boiling water, allowed to steep for 5 minutes, and then ingested. Cinnamon sticks also can be steeped in boiling water to make a tea, and ingested three times daily. Honey can be added to taste. Fresh red and black dates are an old Chinese remedy. Eat several at the end of each meal.

EFFECTIVE CHINESE HERBS

Radix glycyrrhizae • Licorice • *Gan cao*
Traditionally used to replenish qi and remove toxins, while having an antispasmodic effect. Pharmacologically, has anti-inflammatory and antispasmodic effects, as well as an effect of increasing blood pressure.

Ramulus cinnamomi • Cinnamon • *Gui zhi*
Traditionally used to remove obstructions to qi and promote its flow through the channels. Pharmacologically, has tranquilizing and analgesic effects.

Coptidis rhizoma • Coptis • *Huang lian*
Traditionally used to remove toxins and dispel heat. Pharmacologically, lowers the blood pressure.

Gui zhi can cao tang, consisting of:
Radix glycyrrhizae (Gan cao) 5 g.
Ramulus cinnamomi (Gui zhi) 10 g.

Hypothyroidism

DEFINITION A disorder in which there is decreased activity or functioning of the thyroid.

SYMPTOMS Characterized by lethargy, fatigue, edema, or swelling, coldness in the extremities, slowness, frequent urination, avoidance of cold, and above normal weight with normal eating patterns.

NATURAL FOOD REMEDIES

The herb *Coleus forskohlii* increases thyroid production. Available as an extract, it should be taken under the direction of a physician.

Both fennel and pepper are reported to have benefits for hypothyroidism. An effective tea can be made from the fronds of fennel mixed with 1/8 teaspoon of cayenne pepper and an equal amount of nutmeg. Combine with 2 cups of boiling water, allow the mixture to steep for 5 minutes and then strain. Take twice daily.

Walnuts and pistachio nuts, both easily added to salads, are reported to enhance blood pressure. A Chinese natural food remedy is kidneys, which should be sliced, cooked with rice, and eaten daily.

EFFECTIVE CHINESE HERBS

Radix angelicae sinesis • Angelica • *Dang gui*
Traditionally used to move and enhance the blood. Pharmacologically, enhances metabolism while promoting urine excretion.

Eucommiae cortex • Eucommia • *Du zhong*
Traditionally used to aid the liver while strengthening bones.
Pharmacologically, increases the absorption of cholesterol.

Cervicolla cornus • Antler gelatin • *Lu jiao jiao*
Traditionally used for ailments resulting from deficient cold.

Typical Herbal Formula

You gui wan, consisting of:
Radix angelicae sinesis (Dang gui) 80 g.
Eucommia cortex (Du zhong) 100 g.
Cervicolla cornus (Lu jiao jiao) 100 g.
Aconiti tuber (Fu zi) 50 g.
Cortex cinnamomi (Gui pi) 50 g.
Dioscoreae bulbiferae rhizoma (Huang yao zi) 100 g.
Corni fructus (Shan zhu yu) 80 g.
Radix rehmanniae praeparatae (Shou di huang) 200 g.
Cuscutae semen (Tu si zi) 100 g.

Impotence

DEFINITION Lack of copulative power or virility. Impotence can have its origins in a variety of problems, the majority of which are physical, including clogged arteries and secondary effects of medications. Emotional problems or unresolved conflicts can also cause impotence.

SYMPTOMS The inability to have or maintain an erection in spite of an emotional desire to have sexual intercourse.

Natural Food Remedies

Note that the remedies listed here all require ingestion for several weeks before results may be realized.

When arteriosclerosis is the causative factor, keep the arteries flowing freely with diet low in fat and high in fiber and fruits. To increase fiber in the diet, red soybeans or soybeans should be added to the diet daily. Although actually a popular dessert in southern China, red soybean soup is an excellent way to ingest soybeans daily. Wash the red soybeans and soak for several hours in cool water. Rinse, add more water, bring the mixture to a boil, and simmer until the beans are soft and of a medium-thick consistency. Garlic and other spices can be added to make a flavorful soup, although the Chinese add sugar to make a sweet, pudding-like mixture that they eat as a cold dessert.

Taken either as an extract daily, a tea, or food additive, ginseng is reported to have beneficial effects for this disorder. Job's tears, also, can be made into a tea by mixing 1 teaspoon of the seeds with 2 cups of boiling water. Let steep for 5 minutes, strain the seeds from the liquid, and take twice daily.

Ginkgo has been found to improve the flow of blood in the vessels of the penis. Available in a variety of forms including tablets and extract, ginkgo should be taken daily in the doses recommended. Royal jelly also, an extract of bee pollen, is available in liquid form and should be ingested daily in the dosage called for on the package.

EFFECTIVE CHINESE HERBS

Ginkgo semen • Ginkgo • *Yin xing*
Traditionally used to improve qi. Pharmacologically, has an antibacterial effect and improves blood flow.

Radix rehmanniae • Rehmannia • *Sheng di huang*
Traditionally used to nourish yin and blood. Pharmacologically, is shown to have cardiotonic and diuretic effects.

TYPICAL HERBAL FORMULA

Zhi bai di huang wan, consisting of:
Radix rehmannia (Shou di huang) 200 g.
Corni fructus (Shan zhu yu) 100 g.
Dioscoreae rhizoma (Shan yao) 100 g.

Rhizoma alismatis (Ze xie) 90 g.
Poria cocos (Fu ling) 80 g.
Radix paeoniae lactiflora (Chi shao) 6 g.
Anemarrhena asphodeloides (Zhi mu) 80 g.
Phellodendri cortex (Huang bo) 80 g.

Insomnia

DEFINITION A disorder in which the individual suffers from an inability to sleep. Causes are numerous and include increased caffeine intake, secondary effects of medications, stress, change in sleep time, emotional problems, secondary effects of food intake, and secondary effects of other ailments.

SYMPTOMS An inability to fall asleep with frequent tossing and turning, awakening easily or with no reason after falling asleep, nervousness, irritability, fatigue, poor appetite, disturbing dreams, periods of anxiety, and diminished functioning.

NATURAL FOOD REMEDIES

Investigate any changes in diet, medications, or habits. Consider a diet low in fats, and high in carbohydrates, fiber, and fruit. Carbohydrates naturally raise the blood sugar level, causing one to feel sleepy. Dates, for examples, are high in sugar; eating 20 to 30 grams as a bedtime snack induces sleep.

A hot, soothing drink before bedtime can also bring on sleep. The perennial plant valerian has a mild sedative action and is available in a variety of forms. Steep 1 tablespoon of the dried root in 2 cups of boiling water for 5 minutes, add honey to taste, and take 45 minutes before retiring. Honey alone can be make a soothing drink by adding a cup of boiling water and lemon and ingesting 45 minutes prior to bedtime. Another tea can be made with 30 to 40 grams of lily flowers boiled in water and sweetened with honey.

Chamomile tea, made from the plant *Matricaria chamomilla*, is known to have a calming effect. Add a teaspoon of the dried flowers to 1 cup of boiling water and allow to steep 5 minutes before sipping. Finally, the common oat is available as a tincture and has a calming effect. Add 10 drops to tepid water and take an hour before bedtime.

EFFECTIVE CHINESE HERBS

Rhizoma cnidii • Cnidium • *Chuan xiong*
Traditionally used to encourage the flow of qi while improving blood circulation. Pharmacologically, has hypotensive and vasodialating effect while acting as an antispasmodic.

Rhizoma pinelliae • Pinellia • *Ban xia*
Traditionally used to remove dampness, accumulations, and swelling while soothing the stomach. Pharmacologically, has antiemetic and sedative effects.

Radix ginseng • Ginseng • *Ren shen*
Traditionally used to calm the internal spirit while promoting qi. Pharmacologically, increases the resistance of the body to stress by acting on the pituitary gland.

Zizyphi spinosi semen • Jujube seed • *Suan zao ren*
Traditionally used to soothe the spirit and heart while reinforcing yin. Pharmacologically, has a sedative effect, inhibiting the central nervous system, while also a hypotensive effect.

TYPICAL HERBAL FORMULA

Yang xin tang, consisting of:
Thujae orientalis semen (Bo zi ren) 5 g.
Rhizoma pinelliae (Ban xia) 15 g.
Rhizoma cnidii (Chuan xiong) 15 g.
Radix angelicae sinesis (Dang gui) 15 g.
Poria cocos (Fu ling) 15 g.

Hoelen (Fu shen) 5 g,
Radix glycyrrhizae (Gan cao) 5 g.
Radix astragali (Huang qi) 15 g.
Radix ginseng (Ren shen) 8 g.
Ramulus cinnamomi (Gui zhi) 3g.
Zizyphi spinosi semen (Suan zao ren) 8 g.
Fructus schizandrae (Wu wei zi) 8 g.
Radix polygalae (Yuan zhi) 8 g.

Intestinal Parasites

DEFINITION A disorder in which the intestines are inhabited by parasitic organisms. Although more frequently encountered in countries where drinking water is infested and food sources unmonitored, because of increasing world travel, it is not uncommon anywhere. Frequently, travelers find themselves with irritable bowel syndrome and leave the ailment untreated until more serious symptoms appear. If you develop gastro-intestinal symptoms after eating raw vegetables or suspect food, drinking non-potable water, or travel abroad, you should suspect this disorder.

SYMPTOMS These include nausea, vomiting, diarrhea, general abdominal discomfort, malaise, loss of appetite, anal itching, and foul-smelling stools. Accurate diagnosis is made by microscopic evidence.

NATURAL FOOD REMEDIES

Pomegranate is an effective treatment in parasitic infections. One can simply extract the juice from a ripe pomegranate and add a clove of crushed garlic. Add honey or sugar to taste and ingest 6 ounces of this liquid twice daily for fourteen consecutive days. For world travelers, this treatment can be instituted as a preventative measure.

Papaya is also an effective treatment in parasitic infections. The ripe papaya fruit should be eaten at least twice daily for seven consecutive days. A delicious and effective drink can be made by blending papaya with mango and adding a tablespoon of brown sugar. This can be substituted for the raw fruit; however, the effective agent is the papaya, so the quantity of papaya should not be reduced because mango is added.

Coconut is also used to treat parasitic infections. Simply drain the coconut milk into a food processor and process with the fleshy meat of the coconut. Six ounces should be taken for four consecutive days. Coconut candy or dried coconut used for cakes cannot be substituted.

EFFECTIVE CHINESE HERBS

Granati pericarpium • Pomegranate • *Shi liu pi*
Traditionally used to kill intestinal parasites. Pharmacologically, has an antibacterial effect.

Carica papaya • Papaya • *Mu gua*
Traditionally used to relieve fire and create harmony in the stomach. Pharmacologically, is antispasmodic and antibacterial.

Irritable or Nervous Bowel

DEFINITION Cramps or bowel distress commonly known as irritable or spastic colon, a diagnosis typically reached after all others have been ruled out. This disorder is apparently one with which some are afflicted and some are not, and occurs more frequently to sensitive or nervous individuals, usually following meals. In any case, if blood appears in the stool or if bowel symptoms appear suddenly to one who has not had a history of nervous bowel, an immediate medical investigation is warranted, as it may be a symptom of a more serious underlying disorder.

SYMPTOMS Stomach ache, usually following meals, with gas, constipation, and sometime diarrhea. Cramps are the most common symptom, accompanied by tenderness in the abdomen.

Sufferers of an irritable bowel must alter their dietary habits by restricting their fat intake, intake of meats, dairy products, spicy foods, and foods with additives. Fast foods are an absolute irritant. Meals should centered around easily digestible foods such as rice, greens, and potatoes. When the bowel irritation has subsided, other foods can be slowly added but easily digestible foods should remain the foundation of the diet. The natural food of choice for the Chinese who suffer from this disorder is rice. Rice gruel, plain and nourishing, can be supplemented with salted beans for taste. Soybeans, redbeans, and yellow soybeans can be taken in place of rice and all can be supplemented by greens such as Chinese chives, Chinese broccoli, and Chinese kale. Avoid cabbage if it causes you gas and avoid laxatives, which will only further irritate your bowel.

When the stomach is acutely irritated, tofu should be taken twice daily. It can be flavored with fruits such as mango or coconut. Simply place a half mango with a eight ounces of tofu and blend until smooth. Add gelatin and place in a square mold. When cooled, slice into cubes and take twice daily. This dessert of the southern Chinese is not only therapeutic but also delicious.

Propolis, availabe as a tincture, can be taken a half hour before meals. This will provide relief for cramping. Peppermint oil also provides relief in cramping. Take 2 to 4 drops of the oil prior to meals, with water and a slice of bread. Teas of peppermint can be soothing to the stomach. Simply crush several peppermint leaves against the side of a cup with a spoon. Add boiling water and allow to steep for 5 minutes. Add honey to taste.

Another therapeutic tea can be made of chamomile, valerian, and bayberry. All three herbs can be purchased in dry form and also as tinctures. In the dry form, take 1 teaspoon each of chamomile and valerian, 2 teaspoons of bayberry, and add to 6 cups of boiling water. Allow to steep for 10 minutes and then strain. Sip a cup at least three times a day.

If you suffer from a nervous bowel you likely are sensitive or often on edge. You should enhance your suseptibility to bowel trouble by drinking excessive coffee or alcohol, or smoking. Instead of brooding, take a walk or make other efforts to be more active.

Menthae herba • Peppermint • *Bo he*
Traditionally used to disperse wind and heat. Pharmacologically, acts to inhibit intestinal movement.

Laryngitis

DEFINITION: The larynx is the organ which enables one to speak, the so-called voice box. In this disorder, the larynx becomes inflamed, usually from overuse, heavy smoking, or a bacterial or viral infection. People who contract laryngitis typically have repeated episodes and therefore should make every effort to institute treatment once they feel that an episode is oncoming.

SYMPTOMS Sore throat, cough, dryness in the mouth, and sometimes fever that usually results in sudden loss of the voice.

NATURAL FOOD REMEDIES

Evaluate your life style. If you find that your laryngitis comes with overuse of your voice, such as through a habit of shouting, try to change your communication methods; if you are exposed to irritants, try to avoid or remove them.

An effective tea can be made by mixing together 1/8 teaspoon of cayenne pepper with the juice of one lemon and two tablespoons of honey. Mix with a cup of hot water and sip. Peppermint is also soothing and provides relief. Crush several leaves against the side of a cup and add hot water and honey to taste.

Fresh ginger slices can be covered with honey and then sucked, providing relief to the throat. A tea can also be made by steeping the slices in boiling water and ingesting three to four times daily.

The herb yerba santa is available in leaf form. Place 1 teaspoon of the leaves in 4 cups of boiling water and allow to steep for 10 minutes. Strain, add lemon, and take a half cup three times daily.

Echinacea works best if your laryngitis is due to a bacterial or viral infection, as it has anti-inflammatory and antibacterial properties. Make a drink by steeping 1 teaspoon of the dried herb in 2 cups of boiling water. Strain and take three times a day.

Singers, or anyone whose who laryngitis is related to overuse or strain of the throat, should make an echinacea throat spray and use it daily. Combine a teaspoon each of echinacea, red sage, and chamomile in a cup of water that has been boiled and cooled. Place in an atomizer and spray the back of the throat at least four times each day.

EFFECTIVE CHINESE HERBS

Folium perillae • Perilla leaf • *Zi su ye*
Traditionally used to encourage movement of qi while dispelling heat. Pharmacologically, has antibacterial and antipyretic effects.

Semen armeniacae amarcum • Apricot Seed • *Xing ren*
Traditionally used to reduce cough while aiding moisture to lungs. Pharmacologically, an antitussive.

Radix peucedani • Peucedanum • *Qian hu*
Traditionally used to disperse wind and heat, while reducing phlegm. Pharmacologically, has an antihistamine action and causes secretion of fluids in the bronchii.

TYPICAL HERBAL FORMULA

Xing su san, consisting of:
Citri endocarpium (Ju bai) 6g.
Rhizoma pinelliae (Ban xia) 10 g.
Poria cocos (Fu ling) 10 g.
Radix glycyrrhizae (Gan cao) 2 g.
Folium perillae (Zi su ye) 6 g.
Semen armeniacae amarcum (Xing ren) 9 g.
Radix peucedani (Qian hu) 6 g.
Radix platycodi (Jie geng) 6 g.
Fructus jujubae (Da zao) 6 g.

Leg Cramps

DEFINITION Tenderness or pain the legs, particularly cramping, with resultant impaired ability to ambulate. This occurs only when ambulating and has its origins in disturbed blood flow, and is also known as claudication, or spasm of the blood vessels in the legs. It can be extremely painful to the sufferer and episodes can occur quite suddenly, particularly in cold, damp weather.

SYMPTOMS Leg pain, cramps, limping with increasing severity while ambulating.

NATURAL FOOD REMEDIES

The diet should be altered to decrease the fat and meat intake while increasing intake of fruits and green leafy vegetables. A particularly healthful drink can be made by combining bok choy and Chinese broccoli or Chinese spinach in equal amounts and extracting the juices, with 6 ounces taken at least twice daily.

Gingko increases the circulation and is particularly effective for circulatory diseases. A tincture can easily be added to the juice described above. It should be taken on a regular basis since this disorder requires continued treatment to be effective.

Blackstrap molasses, high in B complex vitamins, has been reported to be effective. Add 1 tablespoon to 1 cup of boiling water, allow to cool, and then sip. Take after rising and then twice daily. Hawthorn berries also relieve circulatory difficulty. Available as an extract, 10 drops three times daily provides relief.

Chestnuts are an old Chinese remedy to improve circulation in the legs, and can be eaten raw daily.

EFFECTIVE CHINESE HERBS

Ginko semen • Ginko • *Yin xing*
Traditionally used to increase flow of qi. Pharmacologically, increases blood flow.

Crataegi fructus • Hawthorn • *Shan zha*
Traditionally utilized to resolve accumulation. Pharmacologically, has a vasodilative effect.

Menopause

DEFINITION   This condition is a natural cessation of menstrual bleeding in the female, usually occurring between the ages of 46 and 56. During the menopausal period, there is an increase in follicle-stimulating hormones, as the body attempts to stimulate the ovaries to produce estrogen. However, this is the time in the life of the of a female that the ability to bear children ceases. Commonly called the change of life, it can indeed be a time of physical and emotional disruption in the female, as great discomfort can accompany alterations in hormonal production.

SYMPTOMS   Menopausal syndrome is characterized by so-called hot flashes (paroxysmal sweating and flushing), palpitations, vaginal and skin dryness, edema, inability to concentrate, stress incontinence, and feelings of depression, fatigue, irritability, and anxiety. The most serious symptom of menopause is osteoporosis. Emotionally, it is a volatile period with wide mood swings.

NATURAL FOOD REMEDIES

Phytoestrogens are plant estrogens that have a structure similar to estrogens. Foods high in phytoestrogens should become the mainstays of the diet with fats and meats restricted. These foods include soybeans, soybean products, nuts, cereals, whole wheat, grains (excluding white rice), eggplant, peppers, tomatoes, and fruits such as cherries and apples. By increasing the intake of phytoestrogens, the body is fooled into "thinking" that estrogen levels are higher than they actually are. Those who alter their diet in this manner should have a less traumatic menopause.

Try any recipes that substitute tofu for meat products. For instance, try an egg salad which substitutes firm tofu for eggs. Simply mix a tablespoon of fat-free mayonnaise with chopped onion, green pepper, and 6 ounces of firm tofu that has been lightly crushed. Mix and serve on a toasted bagel. Or, try a simple broth made of a vegetable cube and three cups of boiling water. Add a bit of chopped scallion, a chopped herb of your choice (try cilantro), and some tofu cubes.

An old Chinese remedy to calm nervousness and decrease palpitations, as well as regulate the bowels, is to ingest 30 grams of red dates daily.

Agnus castus, the herb of the chaste tree, is a well known treatment for menopause in the United Kingdom and Europe. It is conveniently available in tablets and in tincture form and is highly effective in relief of menopausal mood swings and hot flashes. Simply follow the directions of the form which you are taking with a five-day break between dosage periods, to simulate a normal menstrual cycle.

The herb black cohosh (*Cimicifuga racemosa*) is known to normalize the female system and offers relief in cases of painful menstruation. It is available both in dried form and also as a tincture. Steep 1 teaspoon of the dried root in 2 cups of boiling water. Allow to steep until room temperature and then take a cup three times a day.

Another treatment for hot flashes is to replace coffee and alcoholic drinks with 8 ounces of a juice made of equal amounts of Chinese broccoli or bok choy, combined with juices of beet, celery, and parsley.

Twice daily doses of 30 milliliters of cuttlefish ink provide relief in emotional volatility. Night sweats can be decreased in frequency by sipping 1 cup three times daily of a tea made by adding several cinnamon twigs to 4 cups of boiling water and steeping. Another remedy for night sweats is aloe, 1 teaspoon crushed and taken with warmed honey and water.

Finally, mink and ground oyster shell powder provide the calcium that the body needs during this period. These can be mixed with one of the above juices to be made more palatable.

Radix angelicae sinensis • Angelica • Dang gui
Traditionally used to nourish blood and promote circulation. Pharmacologically, acts to regulate menstruation and menstrual clamping.

Polygoni multiflori caulis • Fleece flower • *Ye jiao teng*
Traditionally used to strengthen meridians and nourish blood. Pharmacologically, has a tranquilizing effect.

Radix rehmanniae praeparata • Prepared rehmannia • *Shou di huang*
Traditionally used to tone and supplement the blood and liver. Pharmacologically, has a diuretic effect.

Testudinis plastrum • Tortoise shell • *Gui pan*
Traditionally used as a blood supplement and to nourish yin. Pharmacologically, has an analgesic effect.

TYPICAL HERBAL FORMULAS

Liu wei di huang wang (when the symptoms are primarily irregular menses, palpitations, anxiety, weakness, night diaphoresis, and flushing in the face), consisting of:

Radix paeonia alba (Bai shao) 10 g.
Poria cocos (Fu ling) 10 g.
Rhizoma alismatis (Ze xie) 10 g.
Dioscorea alata (Shan yao) 10 g.
Fructus corni (Shan zhu yu) 5 g.
Radix *rehmannia praeparata (Shou di huang)* 10 g.

Gui pi tang (when symptoms are primarily delayed or painful menses, severe hot flashes, anxiety, depression, fear, or insomnia), consisting of:

Radix codonopsis (Dang shen) 10 g.
Rhizoma atractylodes (Bai zhu) 8 g.

Poria cocos (Fu ling) 10 g.
Radix astragalus (Huang qi) 10 g.
Radix glycyrrhiza (Gan cao) 3 g.
Radix angelica dahuricae (Bai zhi) 5 g.
Fructus jujubae (Da zao) 10 g.
Polygala tenuifolia (Yuan zhi) 5g.
Radix saussurea (Mu xiang) 5 g.
Zingiberis sciccatum rhizoma (Gan jiang) 5 g.

Morning Sickness

DEFINITION   A common problem during pregnancy, characterized by nausea and vomiting in the morning during the first trimester of pregnancy due to a change in hormonal levels. If it occurs to great severity, dangerous dehydration can result.

SYMPTOMS Nausea, vomiting, loss of appetite, and general malaise without fever or other signs of infection; dehydration when severe.

NATURAL FOOD REMEDIES

Ginger root has a dramatic effect in soothing the stomach and counteracting nausea. A soothing tea is easily made by adding several slices of ginger to 2 cups of boiling water and steeping for 3 to 5 minutes. Remove the ginger, and add honey to taste, and sip slowly several times daily.

A Chinese folk remedy is a watery rice gruel to which is added several slices of ginger. Bring to a boil 1/4 cup of rice in 6 cups of water and then simmer until the rice grains break down. Add water to keep the fluid level constant, and add several slices of ginger during the last half hour of cooking. With a touch of honey and cinnamon, the mixture can be taken as breakfast food to quell the stomach.

It is helpful to reduce your fat intake while the stomach is sensitive. Eat toast or crackers with your tea, without butter.

Chew one or two leaves of feverfew a day for relief from nausea. Or take twice daily a tea made by steeping a teaspoon of the herb in 1 cup of boiling water. Mint tea also can sooth the stomach and prevent nausea. It is easily made by crushing several leaves against the side of a cup with a spoon and adding hot water. Allow to steep for several minutes and then sweeten and sip, three times daily. The mint tea can be combined with ginger.

EFFECTIVE CHINESE HERBS

Radix pulsatillae • Pulsatilla • *Bai tou wen*
Traditionally used to cool the blood and dispel heat. Pharmacologically, has an antibacterial effect and is a vasodilator.

Strychni semen • Nux vomica • *Ma qian zi*
Traditionally used to remove fluids and move meridians while soothing the spirit. Pharmacologically, stimulates the central nervous system and increases intestinal peristalsis.

Motion Sickness

DEFINITION Commonly known as sea sickness or air sickness, motion sickness is a disturbance of the inner ear caused by movement of the body, resulting in nausea and dizziness.

SYMPTOMS Nausea, vomiting, and dizziness, with an increase in symptoms upon experiencing unpleasant odors accompanied by a feeling of spinning or being off balance.

NATURAL FOOD REMEDIES

Feverfew leaves can be eaten but are extremely bitter. In preparation for a boat ride or similar trip where motion sickness might be experienced, try a feverfew tea. Steep several leaves in 2 cups of hot water, strain, flavor with honey or lemon, and drink at least an hour before your trip.

Ginger is a great stomach settler. Try ginger tea or coat several slices with honey and suck on them. Take some slices along on your trip and suck on a slice or two when you experience discomfort.

Licorice is available as a tincture. Place 4 or 5 drops in a glass of carrot juice and add a slice of pulverized ginger. Take 6 ounces at least one hour prior to your trip.

EFFECTIVE CHINESE HERBS

Rhizoma atractylodis • Atractylodes • *Bai zhu*
Traditionally used to tone the qi and settle the stomach. Pharmacologically, promotes digestion and has an antiemetic effect.

Radix codonopsitis • Codonopsitis • *Dang shen*
Traditionally used to move fluids while promoting qi. Pharmacologically, promotes digestion and dilates blood pressure while stimulating the nervous system.

Paralysis (from Stroke)

DEFINITION A cerebral vascular accident, commonly called a stroke, is a serious medical condition in which one of the vessels supplying blood to the brain ruptures or is occluded. The area of the brain supplied by that particular blood vessel is deprived of its nourishment and hence has decreased functioning. One of the prime disabilities is paralysis, or loss of motor function.

SYMPTOMS Loss of motor function in some area of the body. Accompanying this is usually some loss of memory and some disruption of thought processes. The individual often suffers from depression and loss of self esteem.

Ginkgo (*Gankgo biloba*) has demonstrated an ability to increase blood flow to the brain, enhance neural activity, and aid in memory performance. Not only has it been used recently in treatment of those individuals who have suffered cerebral vascular accidents to increase blood flow to the brain but it has also been used preventively. It is now available in tablets, tinctures, and powders, with dosage depending upon the form ; however, it should be taken in even intervals throughout the day.

Ginseng also enhances circulation. It is best taken as a tea and ingested in evenly spaced dosages throughout the day, but it is also available in tablet and tincture form.

Soy lecithin can be obtained in tablet form and should be taken daily. The diet should be enhanced by ingestion of soy products including soybeans and tofu. Increase also the intake of leafy green vegetables. Equal amounts of juices of parsley, Chinese broccoli, lettuce, and celery should be mixed, with 8 ounces taken daily.

Royal jelly, the product of worker bees, improves functioning of the nervous system and promotes circulation and should be taken daily.

EFFECTIVE CHINESE HERBS

Radix rehmanniae praeparata • Prepared rehmannia • *Shou di huang*
Traditionally used for yin deficiency of the blood. Pharmacologically, is a nutrifying agent and promotes diuresis.

Rhizoma alismatis • Alisma • *Ze xie*
Traditionally used to remove dampness by promoting diuresis. Pharmacologically, promotes diureis and has a hypotensive effect.

Dendrobii caulis • Dendrobium • *Shi hu*
Traditionally used to nourishes yin and expel heat. Pharmacologically, has an antipyretic and analgesic effect.

Dendrobii caulis (Shi hu) 10 g.
Radix glycyrrhizae (Gan cao) 5 g.
Radix astragali (Huang qi) 10 g.
Rhizoma alismatis (Ze xie) 10 g.
Asparagi radix (Tian men dong) 10 g.
Radiz ophiopogonis (Mai men dong) 5 g.
Eriobotryae folium (Pi pa ye) 5 g.
Radix ginseng (Ren shen) 10 g.

Pelvic Inflamatory Disease

DEFINITION   An inflammation of the female pelvic organs which may include the vagina, ovaries, pelvic connective tissues, uterus, and fallopian tubes. In most instances, infection is introduced through the vagina which results in a vaginitis or inflammation of the vaginal canal. Infection can quickly spread from the vagina to other areas of the female pelvis.

SYMPTOMS   Vaginal discharge, abdominal pain, and tenderness, fever, distention of the lower abdomen, lumbago, general malaise, and vomiting.

NATURAL FOOD REMEDIES

St. John's wort is available in many forms. As an ointment, it can be applied directly to relieve irritation of the vaginal canal. Pomegranate juice makes an effective douche. Simply crush the pomegranate to extract the juice and mix with an equal amount of water that has been boiled and allowed to cool to room temperature. Douche twice daily with the mixture.

Fenugreek seeds can be infused to make a tea. Steep 1 tablespoon of seeds in 2 cups of boiling water for 5 minutes. Strain, flavor with honey if desired, and take three times daily. Pulsatilla is effective when there is vaginal discharge and temperature. Take three times daily in the suggested dose. Another effective remedy is 20 drops of tincture of echinacea, taken daily mixed with carrot or grapefruit juice.

Garlic also provides positive benefits. Available in natural, pill, or ground form, it is best taken naturally. Simply ingest 3 cloves of garlic three times daily, crushed and added to food, or crushed with honey and eaten.

EFFECTIVE CHINESE HERBS

Houttuyniae herba • Fishwort • *Yu xing cao*
Traditionally used to dissipate heat and treat abscesses. Pharmacologically, has antibacterial, antifungal, and diuretic effects.

Radix scutellariae • Scute • *Huang qin*
Traditionally used to remove heat and fire, as well as to remove toxic elements. Pharmacologically, has antibacterial and antipyretic effects.

TYPICAL HERBAL FORMULA

Radix scutellariae (Huang qin) 10 g.
Houttuyniae herba (Yu xing cao) 15 g.
Lonicerae flos (Jin yin hua) 15 g.
Sargentodoxae caulis (Hong teng) 15 g.
Phellodendri cortex (Huang bo) 10 g.
Radix paeoniae lactiflora (Chi Shao) 10 g.
Rhei rhizoma (Da huang) 10 g.
Radix glycyrrhizae (Gan cao) 10 g.

Peptic Ulcer

DEFINITION   The stomach, esophagus, and intestines are lined with mucous membrane. When the mucous surface loses its ability to repel acids from the stomach, there is erosion of the surface, which results in an ulcer. In layman's terms, the acid in the stomach literally eats the internal surface of the stomach, intestine, or esophagus. Ulcers should always be evaluated by a physician as they could be indicative of other serious ailments.

SYMPTOMS Stomach ache or cramps which improve with ingestion of food or soothing fluids such as milk. When the stomach is empty, symptoms worsen, with indigestion, dysphasia, hiccups, vomiting, vomiting of blood, and the appearance of blood in the feces as tarry stools.

NATURAL FOOD REMEDIES

Reduce intake of foods high in cholesterol such as red meats, fast foods, and foods with additives. Habits that cause stress to the body such as smoking and drinking alcohol or liquids high in caffeine should be curtailed. Bland foods such as rice gruel, soybeans and soybean products, fruits, and leafy green vegetables should supplant meat intake, particularly during acute phases of the disease. It is always easier to alter the diet during the acute phase as there is great pain; however, long term dietary changes are most therapeutic.

During an acute phase, try *juk*, or southern Chinese rice gruel. Bring a cup of round grain rice in a quart of water to a boil, then simmer until the rice breaks down to a thick soup. Flavor with soybeans, a touch of sesame oil, and coriander. It will not only soothe your stomach but with the addition of parsley, it is therapeutic. If it is not to your tasre, try making the mixture without the soybeans, sesame oil, coriander and in their place add a quarter cup of evaporated skim milk, a teaspoon of cinnamon, and a tablespoon of brown sugar sprinkled on top. A sprinkling of peppermint leaves further enhances its effectiveness.

Propolis, a resin gathered by bees, can be obtained as a tincture. It is highly effective in the treatment of ulcers and should be taken three times per day. Active charcoal mixed with a half glass of water and mixed with honey can be soothing and also relieve gas.

To relieve distress from gas, inflammation, and the pain of ulcers, a tea can be made by adding a teaspoon of fenugreek seeds to 2 cups of boiling water, steeping for 5 minutes, straining and taking three times daily. Another therapeutic and soothing tea can be made by adding 2 cups of water to a teaspoon of comfrey root.

Allow to steep and then add the mixture to 2 cups of your favorite chamomile tea. Take 1 cup at least three times a day to which you have added the sweetener of your choice.

Foods of the cabbage family such as Brussels sprouts, red cabbage, bok choy, and green cabbage should be ingested daily. These are best steamed or cooked with small amounts of water until soft. Ginger and soy can be added to taste.

EFFECTIVE CHINESE HERBS

Rhizoma pinelliae • Pinellia • *Ban xia*
Traditionally used to create harmony in the stomach and remove dampness. Pharmacologically, has an antiemetic and sedative effect.

Radix ophiopogonis • Ophiopogon • *Mai men dong*
Traditionally used to remove heat while purifying the yin. Pharmacologically, has an antipyretic and anti-inflammatory effect.

TYPICAL HERBAL FORMULA

Mai men dong tang, consisting of:
Radix ophiopogonis (Mai men dong) 8 g.
Fructus jujubae (Dao zao) 8 g.
Rhizoma pinelliae (Ban xia) 8 g.
Mi (Jing mi) 8 g.
Radix glycyrrhizae (Gan cao) 4 g.

Pneumonia (Walking)

DEFINITION An inflammation of the lung which progresses to a more severe lobar pneumonia. It is usually described as a resistant cold and sometimes the sufferer is not aware that the cold has progressed to a more serious inflammation. Any severe cold which does not respond to treatment should be medically evaluated.

Chronic cough, fever, shortness of breath, general malaise, headache.

Natural Food Remedies

A tea can be made from Job's tears by steeping 1 teaspoon of the seeds in 2 cups of water for 5 minutes and then straining. Take three times daily. Or, a coffee can be made by roasting the seeds in a dry frying pan and then crushing them. Add 2 cups of water and steep for 5 minutes before straining. Drink three times daily.

Equal amounts of celery, orange, and parsley should pulverized, juices extracted, with 6 ounces taken twice daily. Fresh peppermint leaves may also be steeped in hot water for 5 minutes and then strained. Add crushed strawberries, sweeten with honey and take 1 cup three times daily.

A tablespoon of blackstrap molasses can be added to 2 cups of boiling water. Allow to come to room temperature, add lemon juice, and ingest 1 cup twice a day.

Lobelia is an effective expectorant that causes relaxation of the bronchial muscles. It is available as a dried herb, a tincture, or an extract. The dried herb can be infused by mixing a teaspoon with 2 cups of boiling water and steeping for 5 minutes. The mixture is strained and a cup taken three times daily.

Effective Chinese Herbs

Radix puerariae • Pueraria • *Ge gen*
Traditionally used to remove internal heat and nourish the blood vessels. Pharmacologically, is antipyretic and increases blood flow.

Radix peucedani • Peucedanum • *Qian hu*
Traditionally used to dispel wind and heat while moving qi downward. Pharmacologically, acts as an expectorant and antihistamine.

Rhizoma pinelliae • Pinellia • *Ban xia*
Traditionally used to remove moisture while dispersing accumulated moisture. Pharmacologically, has an antiemetic effect.

Rhizoma pinelliae (Ban xia) 5 g.
Radix puerariae (Ge gen) 10 g.
Radix codonopsis (Dang shen) 10 g.
Poria cocos (Fu ling) 10 g.
Folium perillae (Zi Su ye) 5 g.
Radix glycyrrhizae (Gan cao) 5 g.
Radix peucedani (Qian hu) 10 g.

Prostatitis

DEFINITION A disorder of the prostate gland, the gland which surrounds the urethra between the bladder and the penis. When the prostate gland becomes infected and inflamed, it is not uncommon for the infection to extend into the urethra or bladder. However the most common disorder of the prostate gland is benign hypertrophy, simply an enlarged prostate gland. The most serious disorder of the prostate in older males is malignancy of the prostate. Noting the many origins of disorders of the prostate, it is imperative that the causative factor be evaluated.

SYMPTOMS Difficulty in urinating with dribbling and inability to empty the bladder. In addition, there may be pain and swelling upon sitting, fever, chills, blood in the urine, or cloudy urine accompanied by a feeling of a growth between the legs.

Natural Food Remedies

For both prevention and treatment of benign prostatic hypertropy, a diet high in zinc is recommended. One can gain the recommended therapeutic amount of zinc in the diet by eating a half cup of pumpkin seeds daily. These should not be the salted variety as these increase the sodium intake, detrimental to the health for other reasons. Liquids should be increased, with 8 ounces of water drunk at least six to eight times per day. Alcohol intake should be curtailed.

Saw palmetto (*Serenoa serrulata*) is an herb which has had proven positive effects on the prostate. It has a diuretic action in addition to an anti-inflammatory action. One of the most annoying symptoms, frequent night urination, is stemmed by taking this herb. Available in a number of forms, a teaspoon of the berries can be infused with 4 cups of water and allowed to steep for 30 minutes. After the mixture is strained, it should be ingested three times daily.

Cernilton, another flower extract, has actions similar to those of saw palmetto. It has an anti-inflammatory action while relaxing the urethra and has been effective in the treatment of prostatitis. The extract should be taken as directed.

Cornsilk has long been utilized in the treatment of prostatitis. Cornsilk and banana peel should be added to 1 quart of water and brought to a boil. When cooled, the mixture is strained and a cup of the liquid is taken four times a day.

Echinacea, available as a tincture and in a dried form, has an antibacterial effect. A drink can be made by adding a tablespoon of the root to 4 cups of water and bringing to a boil. Steep for 10 minutes, and take a cup three times daily.

It is known that the incidence of prostate disease in Japan is well below that of the West. Many scientists believe that diet plays an important causative role in this and recommend a diet high in vegetable, fiber, and soy products in place of a diet high in meats. Soybean products may not only influence the diet in that it replaces meat products but may also block the growth of blood vessels that feed tumors.

TYPICAL HERBAL FORMULA

Long dan xie gan wan, consisting of:
Rhizoma alismatis (Zi xie) 15 g.
Radix bupleuri (Chai hu) 15 g.
Gentianae radix (Long dan) 16 g.
Radix scutellaria (Huang qin) 7 g.
Akebiae caulis (Mu tong) 7 g.

Plantaginis semen (Che qian zi) 7 g.
Radix angelicae sinensis (Dang gui) 7 g.
Rehmanniae radix (Sheng di huang) 7 g.
Radix glycyrrhizae (Gan cao) 7 g.

Psoriasis

DEFINITION A skin disorder characterized by patches of red, scaly sores usually occurring on the arms, upper torso, scalp, and elbows. The etiology is unknown and there is no known cure. It is not a contagious disorder but it is more apt to occur among members of families where one suffers from the disorder. It is known that persons who suffer from psoriasis are more apt to have episodes when they suffer from emotional stress.

SYMPTOMS Patches of inflamed skin which are red, itchy, flaky, and highly irritating.

NATURAL FOOD REMEDIES

Those whose diet is high in meat content seem to have more episodes of acute psoriasis. It is recommended that meats be restricted from the diet and the diet enhanced with foods high in fiber content. Drink 8 ounces daily of a juice made of equal amounts of beets, Chinese kale, celery, and carrots.

Blackstrap molasses has proven effective in some cases both as a salve and when taken internally. As a salve, the blackstrap molasses mixed with warm water and applied with compresses three to four times daily. At the same time, 1 tablespoon of blackstrap molasses can be mixed with 1 cup of hot water and taken three times daily. Add lemon or lime juice to taste.

Echinacea, commonly known as coneflower, is available in a variety of forms and when taken as prescribed is reported to have positive effects in episodes of psoriasis.

If you feel that your psoriasis is related to tension, try valerian, reported to provide some positive effects when mixed with vervain. Simply mix tinctures of both with your favorite tea, chamomile is recommended, and take three times daily.

For a topical solution, 6 ounces of whole cloves can be mixed with 1 pint of 70 percent alcohol. Allow the solution to remain at room temperature for at least 24 hours, then apply to the infected areas.

Effective Chinese Herbs

Zingiberis rhizoma recens • Fresh ginger • *Sheng jiang*
Traditionally used to remove toxins and revolve surfaces. Pharmacologically, has an antibacterial effect, while its oil stimulates the capillaries.

Caryophylli flos • Cloves • *Ding xiang*
Traditionally used to enhance yang. Pharmacologically, has antibacterial, antiviral, and antifungal effects.

Phillodendri cortex • Aloe • *Lu hui*
Traditionally said to remove heat. Pharmacologically, inhibits ulceration.

Raynaud's Disease

DEFINITION Raynaud's Disease or Raynaud's Syndrome is a condition in which the peripheral blood vessels of the hands and feet are compromised, causing pain, numbness, and the skin to turn a bluish color. In essence, blood fails to flow to the extremities; moreover, when the extremities are suddenly warmed, there is extreme pain. The exact cause of this phenomenon is unclear. Some feel that there is an emotional component while others feel it is a disorder of the blood vessels themselves. Persons who suffer from this disease should avoid exposure to cold temperatures, or at least keep the hands or feet well covered.

Symptoms Occurring particularly during cold and during rapid change in temperature are tingling, pain, numbness, and a bluish cast to the skin of the limbs. The disorder is particularly prevalent among long-term smokers.

Natural Food Remedies

Avoid intake of caffeine or nicotine, which cause constriction of blood vessels, and never place affected areas in hot water. Gingko and hawthorn both have vasodilating effects. Make a therapeutic drink by adding equal amounts of the dried herbs to 2 cups of boiling water, allowing the mixture to steep, and taking three times daily. You can also take a teaspoon of the tincture of each, combine with carrot juice, and ingest twice daily.

Pepper aids circulation and has hot properties. Foods which are supplemented by pepper aid circulation and should be eaten regularly. A tonic can be made by mixing hot water with cayenne pepper. Add honey and lemon juice to taste.

Molasses is reported to have had beneficial results, adding 1 teaspoon per cup of any warm, nutritive drink such as tea and drinking at least twice daily. Ginkgo also has been reported to improve circulation. Available in a variety of forms, 100 milligrams should be taken daily.

Effective Chinese Herbs

Radix pulsatillae • Pulsatilla • *Bai tou wen*
Traditionally used to remove toxins. Pharmacologically, is a peripheral blood vessel dilator.

Crataegi fructus • Hawthorn • *Shan zha*
Traditionally said to resolve accumulation. Pharmacologically, has a vasodilative action

Skin Irritations

DEFINITION Causes of skin irritation are many, including the bites of bees or mosquitoes, abrasions, minor burns, and irritations from plants such as poison ivy. All can cause an immediate reaction in the skin, such as swelling, redness, irritation, itching, and in some cases, pain. In severe cases there can be a systemic reaction by the body such as development of a fever, dizziness, difficulty in breathing, or irregular heartbeat. In such cases, immediate medical attention is warranted.

SYMPTOMS Primary symptoms are itching, erythema, or redness, minor swelling, and localized pain.

NATURAL FOOD REMEDIES

St. John's wort, the herb which has found to have remarkable benefits in treatment of depression and anxiety, I have found also to be a treatment for minor wounds and burns. A remedy can be easily made by crushing the flowers and leaves very finely with a mortar and pestle. Place about 3 tablespoons of the mixture in a sterilized jar, add a cup and a half of Vaseline, mix thoroughly, and allow to stand at least 2 days. Keep in the refrigerator so that it is readily available for bites, scrapes, or burns. Apply three times a day to affected areas.

Clean the surface of any abrasion immediately with fresh lemon juice. Pat the surface dry and then squeeze the lemon skin so some of its oils spray on to the abraded surface. Keep dry. In cases of abrasion that do not bleed or break the skin, crush a small piece of aloe, exposing the fleshy substance, and apply it gently to the damaged surface several times a day to expedite healing. Surprisingly, cayenne pepper and crushed Szechuan pepper will bring relief from pain when applied directly to the surface of an abrasion in which the skin is unbroken. After 10 minutes, brush off lightly and keep dry.

When bitten by an insect, immediately remove the stinger and apply tincture of myrrh. This will reduce the swelling and cool the wound. Apply three times daily. Or, crush a bit of papaya and after the stinger has been removed, coat the surface of the wound with the papaya. Apply three times daily. Or, pulverize cilantro and mix with a bit of Vaseline, applying the mixture directly to the surface of the bite.

At the same time, mix one part cilantro, two parts celery, and one part carrots. Pulverize and extract the juice. Take 6 ounces at least twice during the first day following the bite.

For other skin irritations, cleanse the irritated surface immediately with rice vinegar and then air dry. Repeat at least four times daily. Echinacea is available in tablets, and can be taken daily as indicated on the package. Comfrey (*Symphytum officinale*) also, can be obtained in a variety of forms including a powder that can be applied directly to the irritated surface in a mix of one part comfrey and one part cornstarch. Apply immediately and three times daily.

Make a compress of black tea leaves by soaking the leaves in hot water, allowing to cool, and then applying directly to the irritated area.

Finally, crush marigold petals, mix with a small amount of Vaseline or rice vinegar, and apply liberally three times a day. Use Vaseline when the irritation is dry and crusting, and rice vinegar when the area is seeping.

EFFECTIVE CHINESE HERBS

Commiphora myrrha • Myrrh • Mo yao
Traditionally used through the liver meridian to remove swelling and fluids, and increase circulation. Pharmacologically, acts as an antiseptic.

Sore Throat

DEFINITION A sensation of rawness and pain in the throat that is usually sudden in onset and often a sign of impending upper respiratory distress such as a cold or laryngitis. However, it can also be caused by irritation from allergies, or exposure to smoke or chemicals.

SYMPTOMS A sensation of sandpaper-like irritation at the back of the throat, experienced particularly when swallowing, redness in the throat, swelling, and cough. When there is a persistent sore throat, fever, or sore throat unaccompanied by upper respiratory symptoms, medical attention should be sought.

Natural Food Remedies

At the first sign of a sore throat, crush 2 medium-sized cloves of garlic in a small bowl, add a tablespoon of honey or molasses and a bit of fresh lemon juice, and take three times daily. Tumeric mixed with an equal amount of salt in a cup of warm water is an effective gargle. Simply mix and stir until the salt is dissolved, and gargle three times daily.

Place 1 or 2 teaspoons of slippery elm bark bark in 4 cups of water, boil and then simmer for 15 minutes. Drink a cup of the liquid three times daily.

Licorice is available both in root form and as a tincture and makes an effective and soothing tea. Add 5 drops of the tincture to a cup of boiling water with a teaspoon of sugar or honey. Sip a cup three times daily.

Increase your vitamin C intake at the first sign of a sore throat. Recent studies show that the most effective juice is grapefruit juice. Squeeze 8 ounces of grapefruit juice, add a teaspoon of honey, and take twice daily.

EFFECTIVE CHINESE HERBS

Curcumae tuber • Tumeric • *Yu jin*
Traditionally used to control pain while dissolving qi stagnation. Pharmacologically, has an analgesic effect and increases salivation.

Allii bulbus • Garlic • *Da suan*
Traditionally used to aid in the removal of phlegm and promote removal of fluids. Pharmacologically, has antibacterial and antifungal effects.

Stomach Ache

DEFINITION Gastritus, commonly known as stomach ache, is an inflammation of the stomach with a variety of causes, ranging from eating irritating foods to more serious disorders such as malignancies, or cardiac or liver disease. In most instances, the sufferer is aware of the relationship between overindulging and gastritis; however, it is not uncommon for cardiac problems to be masked by epigastric and gastric distress. Noting this, one should always look to the origins of the discomfort and not treat any chronic gastric pain by palliative medicine without investigation.

SYMPTOMS Sudden loss of appetite, nausea, epigastric pain, vomiting, and distention of the stomach, frequently accompanied by cramps and belching. The herbal remedies here are for mild gastritis resulting from irritation from food, as well as preventatives for chronic gastritis.

NATURAL FOOD REMEDIES

Evaluate your diet. In most instances, gastritis is caused from irritants to the stomach, whether from overeating or eating foods highly spiced or high in fats. Simply removing the irritant can be itself a remedy. An old Chinese therapy, equivalent to mother's chicken soup, is *juk*, or rice gruel. Simply combine 1 cup of short-grain rice with 1 quart of water and simmer until the rice has broken down. Flavor with ginger or garlic and a bit of soy for a Chinese-style gruel, or some condensed milk and a touch of cinnamon and nutmeg.

Ginger, sliced and steeped in boiling water, makes a tea which should be ingested at least three to four times daily. It soothes the stomach and promotes relaxation of the smooth muscle.

One teaspoon each of spearmint and peppermint boiled in 1 cup of water and steeped for 10 minutes makes a soothing tea, while a teaspoon of honey helps the taste. A cup at least three times a day is recommended.

Thoroughly dry and pulverize 5 grams of eggshells, and mix with a bland liquid such as diluted tea or hot water. This mixture should be ingested three times daily. Frequently the mixture is combined with ginger.

For gastritus related to colds, try slightly unripe papaya, seeded and pulverized in a blender, with 500 grams eaten twice daily. Honey or brown sugar can be added to taste. Mandarin orange powder or peel makes an effective tea. To 1 gram of powder add 1 cup of boiling water. Sweeten to taste and take at least three times daily.

Effective Chinese Herbs (Overindulgence)

Massa medicinalis fermentata • Medicinal leaven • *Shen gu*
Traditionally used to promote qi and digestion. Pharmacologically, aids in digestive action.

Poria cocos • Hoelen • *Fu ling*
Traditionally used to soothe the "middle warmer" and the nerves while promoting diuresis and relaxing the stomach. Pharmacologically, is a diuretic and has a relaxing effect on the smooth muscles of the stomach.

Raphanus sativa • Radish • *Lai fu zi*
Traditionally used to help qi to descend and encourage digestion. Pharmacologically, acts on the stomach digestive glands and promotes digestion.

Typical Herbal Formula

Bao he wan, consisting of:
Raphanus sativa (Lai fu zi) 10 g.
Poria cocos (Fu ling) 10 g.
Massa medicata fermentata (Shen gu) 10 g.
Crataegi fructus (Shan zha) 10 g.
Fructus forsythiae (Lian qiao) 10g.
Rhizoma pinelliae (Ban xia) 10 g.
Pericarpium papaveris (Chen pi) 10 g.

Alpiniae officinarum rhizoma • Lesser galangal • *Liang jiang*
Traditionally used to expel cold and relieve pain in the stomach.
Pharmacologically, has an analgesic effect.

Rhizoma zingiberis recens • Fresh ginger • *Sheng jiang*
Traditionally used to warm the stomach and control emesis. Pharmacologically, stimulates gastric functioning.

TYPICAL HERBAL FORMULA

Alpiniae officinarum rhizoma (Liang jiang) 10 g.
Zingiberis rhizoma (Sheng jiang) 10 g,
Cyperi rhizoma (Xiang fu zi) 10 g.
Folium perillae (Zi su ye) 5 g.
Evodiae fructus (Wu zhu yu) 5 g.

Urinary Stones

DEFINITION Urinary stones are bits of calcium which crystallize in the urine and can appear in the kidney, the ureter, the tube which extends from the kidney to the bladder, and the bladder itself. These tiny bits of calcium are like bits of grit, and can cause excruciating pain and irritation. Once the small "stones" have formed, it is necessary for the body to rid itself of them. Medical attention is warranted both to confirm the diagnosis but also to evaluate the method of removal.

SYMPTOMS One of the first symptoms is sudden excruciating pain in the back, shoulder, groin, or testicles. There is burning upon urination with blood in the urine and the onset is both sudden and gripping.

The Chinese are not normally water drinkers and therefore, when liquids in the diet are increased, it is usually in the form of tea. Tea intake should be increased to double the normal intake.

Studies reveal that there is a corrolation between urinary stones and diets low in greens and fibers but high in meat products. Changing dietary habits and increasing greens and fibers can reduce the calcium in the urine.

Green vegetables such as Chinese kale, Chinese broccoli. and Chinese chives should be eaten daily, lightly cooked with tofu. Mung bean sprouts and soy products should also be part of the daily diet. Decrease the amount of meat in your diet and increase the amount of fish.

Parsley piert, not to be confused with regular parsley, has been used effectively in treatment of kidney stones. It is available as an extract as well as a dry herb. If you obtain the extract, mix 1 teaspoon with 8 ounces of cranberry juice and take twice daily. Cranberry juice alone is also thought to reduce the amount of calcium in your urine.

EFFECTIVE CHINESE HERBS

Rehmanniae radix • Rehmannia • *Sheng di huang*
Traditionally used to nourish yin and the blood while removing heat. Pharmacologically, has a diuretic effect.

Akebiae Caulis • Akebia • *Mu tong*
Traditionally used to promote blood circulation and movement of water while removing heat. Pharmacologically, has a diuretic effect

TYPICAL HERBAL FORMULA

Dao chi san, consisting of:
Akebiae caulis (Mu tong) 10 g.
Rehmanniae radix (Sheng di huang) 20 g.
Radix glycyrrhizae (Gan cao) 6 g.
Folium bambusae (Zhu ye) 6 g.

Vaginal Infections

DEFINITION Vaginitis is an infection of the vaginal canal which can be induced from tampons, deodorants, douches, condoms, and improper wiping of the anal area. Left untreated, vaginitis can expand into more serious disorders of the pelvic area.

SYMPTOMS Discomfort in the vaginal is usually accompanied by itching, burning, and discharge. The infection can be accompanied by an infection in the bladder.

NATURAL FOOD REMEDIES

St. John's wort relieves the irritation of vaginitis. It is available in a cream and can be applied as directed. However, the best remedy for vaginitis is to prevent its most common cause. After defecating and wiping away from the vaginal area, simply take a clean piece of tissue and moisten with rice vinegar (taking care not to touch the bottle to the tissue) and cleanse the area between the vagina and rectum by wiping backward. Rice vinegar should also be used as a douche for prevention of vaginal infections. Simply mix equal amounts of warm water with rice vinegar for an effective douche.

One ounce of pomegranate flowers (*Punica granatum*) can be mixed with 4 cups of water, brought to a boil. Strained and cooled, the mixture can be bottled in a sterilized jar and utilized as a douche twice daily when a vaginitis is present.

For yeast infections, fill the bottom of the tub with warm water and 1 cup of rice wine vinegar. Place a soft towel between the legs and relax in the water for 10 minutes. Dry with a clean soft cotton cloth. Garlic also is reported to have beneficial effects for yeast infections. Several cloves can be added to food, crushed with honey, or made into a garlic tea. Take three times daily.

Cranberry or blackberry juice should be ingested three times daily, 8 ounces each time. Look for products with the highest percentages of pure fruit juices, rather than "cocktails."

Radix pulsatillae • Pulsatilla • *Bai tou wen*
Traditionally used to remove toxins and heat. Pharmacologically, is antibacterial and antiamebic.

Punica granatum • Pomegranate • *Shi liu*
Traditionally used to remove intestinal parasites. Pharmacologically, is antibacterial and antiviral.

Vomiting

DEFINITION An expulsion of the contents of the stomach through the mouth. Vomiting can related to a multitude of ailments, some severe, so an evaluation of the cause of vomiting deserves attention. For example, it is one of the most common symptoms of fever, influenza, and morning sickness accompanying pregnancy. However, it is also one of the first symptoms of a heart attack and carcinomas of the stomach and gastro-intestinal system.

SYMPTOMS Vomiting is a symptom of an underlying ailment, including simple problems such as overeating, having ingested harmful material, colds and influenza, to more serious conditions, such as growth in the stomach or lower esophagus, intestinal obstruction, liver and cardiac disease, and the like. Herbal remedies enumerated here for the less serious ailments; however, even with severe disorders, herbal remedies can offer some relief of symptoms.

NATURAL FOOD REMEDIES

A potent anti-emetic, ginger slices can be added to 2 cups of boiling water and allowed to steep to make a tea. Add honey or sugar to taste and sip 2 to 3 cups when vomiting is acute.

Peppermint also has an anti-emetic action. Simply crush peppermint leaves against the inside of a cup with a spoon and add boiling water. Allow to steep for 5 minutes, add sugar to taste, take 2 to 3 times daily.

Grapefruit juice is a potent source of vitamin C. Replenish the supply lost in vomiting by adding 1 teaspoon of baking soda and 1 tablespoon of honey to 8 ounces of fresh grapefruit juice. Blend with a slice of ginger, and take 8 ounces three times daily at room temperature.

For vomiting brought on by overeating or overindulgence, charcoal powder in boiling water, allowed to cool and ingested slowly relieves gas and bloating. Mix with honey to make more palatable.

Equal amounts of carrot and apple juice to which is added a slice of ginger replenishes liquids. Take 6 ounces twice daily.

Rice gruel with salted soybeans also can be taken to replenish liquids, and supply nourishment while providing soothing relief to the stomach. This is a common Chinese remedy for overindulgence.

Add 10 drops of hawthorn berry extract to 8 ounces of warm water and take three times daily to counteract stomach spasms; it also has a sedative action.

EFFECTIVE CHINESE HERBS (FOR COLDS OR FLU)

Cortex magnoliae • Magnolia bark • *Hou pu*
Traditionally used through the large intestine to move qi. Pharmacologically, promotes digestion by stimulation of the digestive mucosa.

Arecae pericarpium • Areca peel • *Da fu pi*
Traditionally used through the stomach meridian to cause qi to descend and to dispel water. Pharmacologically, contains tannin.

TYPICAL HERBAL FORMULA

Arecae pericarpium (Da fu pi) 10 g.
Aurantii fructus (Zhi ko) 5 g.
Cortex magnoliae (Hou pu) 5 g.
Radix glycyrrhizae (Gan cao) 5 g.
Rhizoma pinelliae (Ban xia) 10 g.
Rhizoma atractyloides (Cang zhu) 10 g.

Radix pulsatilla • Pulsatilla • *Bai tou wen*
Traditionally used to remove toxins from the system while cooling blood through the stomach meridian. Pharmacologically, is an antibacterial and a blood vessel dilator.

Crataegi fructus • Hawthorn • *Shan zha*
Traditionally used to promote the digestion of food through the stomach meridian. Pharmacologically, increases digestive fluids and digestive action.

Rhizoma pinelliae • Pinellia • *Ban xia*
Traditionally used to create harmony in the stomach while removing dampness. Pharmacologically, has both a sedative and anti-emetic effect.

Typical Herbal Formula

Rhizoma pinelliae (Ban xia) 10 g.
Poria cocos (Fu ling) 10 g.
Crataegi fructus (Shan zha) 10 g.
Massa medicata fermentata (Shen gu) 10 g.
Pericarpium citri (Qing pi) 5 g.
Fructus forsythiae (Lian qiao) 10 g.
Raphanus sativa (Lai fu zi) 6 g.

Index of Herbs

Index of Herbs

Pinyin	Latin	Characters
Bai hua she she cao	Oldenlandiae herba	白花蛇舌草
Bai shao	Radix paeoniae alba	白芍
Bai tou weng	Radix pulsatillae	白头翁
Bai zhu	Rhizoma atractylodis	白术
Ban xia	Rhizoma pinelliae	半夏
Ban zhi lian	Scutellariae barbatae herba	半枝莲
Bi ma zi	Ricini semen	蓖麻子
Bing lang	Areca semen	槟榔
Bo he	Menthae herba	薄荷
Bo zi ren	Thujae orientalis semen	柏子仁
Chai hu	Radix bupleuri	柴胡
Che qian zi	Plantaginis semen	车前子
Chen pi	Pericarpium papaveris	陈皮
Chi shao	Radix paeoniae lactiflora	赤芍
Chi xiao dou	Phaseoli semen	赤小豆
Chuan xiong	Rhizoma cnidii	川芎
Cong bai	Allii fistulosi bulbus	葱白
Da fu pi	Arecae pericarpium	大腺皮
Da huang	Rhei rhizoma	大黄
Da suan	Allii bulbus	大蒜
Da zao	Fructus jujubae	大枣
Dang gui	Radix angelicae sinesis	当归
Dang shen	Radix codonopsitis	党参
Di jiao	Thymi serpylli herba	地椒
Di long	Lumbricus	地龙
Du zhong	Eucommiae cortex	杜仲
E shu	Zedoariae rhizoma	莪术
Fang feng	Radix ledebouriellae	防风 (風)
Feng la	Cera flava	蜂蜡
Fu ling	Poria cocos	茯苓
Fu zi	Aconiti tuber	附子
Gan cao	Radix glycyrrhizae	甘草
Gan jiang	Zingiberis sciccatum rhizoma	干姜

Ge gen	Pueraria	葛根
Gou qi zi	Lycii fructus	枸杞子
Gua lou	Trichosanthis fructus	栝楼
Gui pi	Cortex cinnamomi	桂皮
Gui pan	Tortoise shell	龟板
Gui zhi	Ramulus cinnamomi	桂枝
Hai dong pi	Erythrinae cortex	海桐皮
Hei dou	Glycine sojae semen	黑豆
He shou wu	Polygoni multiflori radix	何首乌
He ye	Nelumbinis folium	荷叶
Hong hua	Carthami flos	红花
Hong teng	Sargentodoxae caulis	红藤
Hou pu	Cortex magnoliae officinalis	厚朴
Hu gu	Os tigris	虎骨
Hu lu pa	Trigonellae semen	葫芦巴
Huang bo	Phellodendri cortex	黄蘖
Huang lian	Coptidiis rhizoma	黄连
Huang qi	Radix astragali	黄耆
Huang qin	Radix scutellariae	黄芩
Huang yao zi	Dioscoreae bulbiferae rhizoma	黄药子
Huo xiang	Herba agastachis	霍香
Jiang huo	Rhizoma seu radix	羌活
Jiang pi	Zingiberis exocarpium	姜皮
Jiao mu	Zanthoxyli bungeani semen	椒目
Jie geng	Radix platycodi	桔梗
Jin qian cao	Desmodii herb	金钱草
Jin yin hua	Lonicerae flos	金银花
Jing jie	Herba schizonepetae	荆芥
Ju bai	Citri endocarpium	橘白
Ju hua	Chrysanthemi flos	菊花
Jue ming zi	Cassiae torae semen	决明子
Lai fu zi	Raphanus sativus	莱菔子
Lian qiao	Fructus forsythiae	莲翘
Liang jiang	Alpiniae officinarum rhizoma	良姜
Ling Zhi	Lucid ganoderma	灵芝
Long dan	Gentianae radix	龙胆
Long kui	Solani herba	龙葵
Long yan rou	Longanae arillus	龙眼肉

Lou lu	Radix echinopsis	漏卢
Lu hui	Phellodendri cortex	卢荟
Lu jiao jiao	Cervicolla cornus	鹿角胶
Ma huang	Radix ephedrae	麻黄
Ma lan jin	Wedeliae herba	马兰金
Ma qian zi	Nux vomica	马钱子
Ma yuen	Coix lacryma jobi	薏苡仁
Mai men dong	Radix ophiopogonis	麦门冬
Mang xiao (Pu xiao)	Natrium sulfuricum	芒硝
Mao dong qing	Radix ilicus pubescentis	毛冬青
Mao zhua cao	Ranunculi ternati radix	猫瓜草
Mo yao	Commiphora myrrha	没药
Mu tong	Aristolochiae caulis	木通
Mu xiang	Radix saussureae	木香
Nu Zhen Zi	Ligustri fructus	女贞子
Pi pa ye	Eriobotryae folium	枇杷叶
Pu yin gen	Radix wikstroemiae	埔银根
Qian hu	Radix peucedani	前胡
Qin jiao	Gentianae macrophyllae radix	秦艽
Qing Pi	Pericarpium citri	青皮
Ren dong teng	Lonicerae caulis et folium	忍冬藤
Ren shen	Radix ginseng	人参
Sang bai pi	Mori cortex	桑白皮
Sang Shen	Mori fructus	桑椹
Shan dou gen	Radixophorae subprostratae	山豆根
Shan yao	Dioscoreae rhizome	山药
Shan zha	Crataegi fructus	山楂
Shan zhu yu	Corni fructus	山茱萸
Shang lu	Radix phytolaccae	商陆
She gan	Belamcandae rhizoma	射干
Shen gu	Massa medicinalis fermentata	神麴
Sheng di huang	Rehmanniae radix	生地黄
Sheng jiang	Rhizoma zingiberis recens	生姜
Sheng ma	Cimfuga rhizoma	升麻
Shi hu	Dendrobii caulis	石斛
Shou di huang	Radix rehmanniae praeparata	熟地黄
Shuo zhuo	Sambucudis caulis et folium	蒴
Suan zao ren	Zizyphi spinosi semen	酸枣仁

Tao ren	Persicae semen	桃仁
Tian kui zi	Radix semiaquilegiae	天葵子
Tu si zi	Cuscutae semen	兔丝子
Wu wei zi	Fructus shisandrae	五味子
Wu zhu yu	Evodiae fructus	吴茱萸
Xi xin	Herba asari	细辛
Xiang fu zi	Cyperi rhizoma	香附子
Xie bai	Bulbus allii macrostemi	薤白
Xin yi	Magnoliae flos	辛夷
Xing ren	Semen armeniacae amarcum	杏仁
Xuan shen	Radix scrophulariae	玄参
Yan hu suo	Rhizoma corydalis tuber	延胡索
Yang mei pi	Myricae cortex	杨梅皮
Yi yi ren	Coicis semen	薏苡仁
Yin xing	Ginkgo semen	银杏
Yu jin	Curcumae tuber	郁金
Yu mi xu	Maydis stigmata	玉米须
Yu xing cao	Houttuyniae herba	鱼腥草
Yuan zhi	Radix polygalae	远志
Zhi ko	Auranthii fructus	枳壳
Zhi mu	Anemarrhenae rhizoma	知母
Zhi zi	Fructus citrus tangerina	支子
Zhu ye	Folium bambusae	竹叶
Zhuo Zhuo	Sambucudis caulis et folium	蒴藋
Zi hua ti ting	Violae herba	紫花地丁
Zi su zi	Folium perillae	紫苏子
Zi wan	Radix asteris	紫菀
Ze xie	Rhizoma alismatis	泽泻

The "weathermark" identifies this book as a production of Weatherhill, Inc., publishers of fine books on Asia and the Pacific. Editorial supervision: Ray Furse. Book and cover design: Mariana Canelo. Production supervision: Bill Rose. Chinese typesetting: Birdtrack Press. Printing and binding: R.R. Donnelley. The typeface used is Goudy.